Discover Your Youthful Radiance

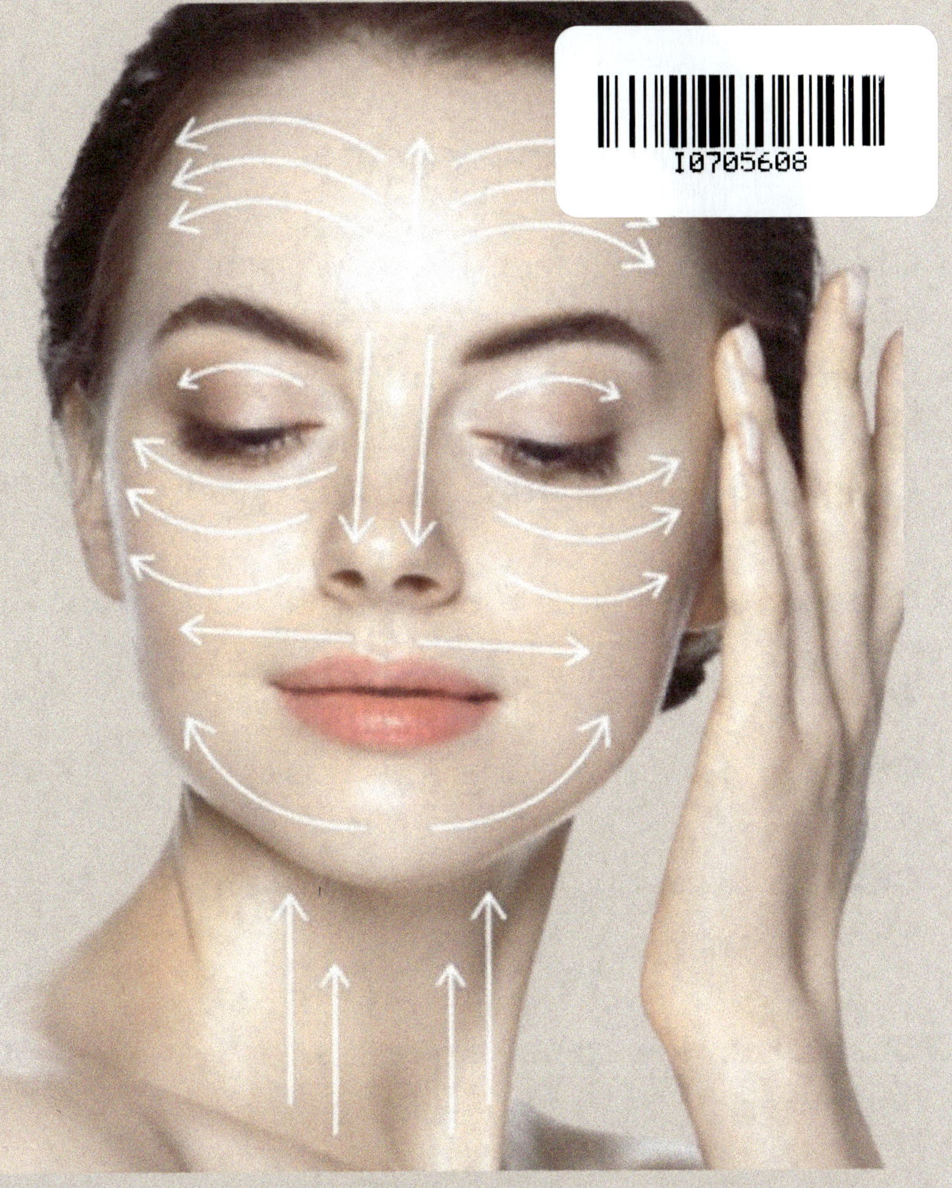

Natural Face Exercises for Novices

TABLE OF CONTENTS

INTRODUCTION

For centuries, the quest for a radiant and youthful appearance has captivated people across cultures. While countless solutions exist, many come with hefty price tags or invasive procedures. But what if there was a natural, accessible approach to sculpting and defining your face?

This book introduces you to the transformative power of face workouts, a simple yet effective way to achieve a more toned and youthful appearance. Forget expensive creams or complicated routines. These exercises utilize the power of your own facial muscles, allowing you to target specific areas and enhance your natural beauty.

The beauty of face workouts lies in their accessibility. No fancy equipment is needed, just your own hands and a few minutes a day. Whether you're a busy professional or someone seeking a natural skincare routine, these exercises can seamlessly fit into your schedule. The best part? The results are cumulative and noticeable. With consistent practice, you'll see improved skin tone, a reduction in fine lines, and a more sculpted appearance – all achieved through the power of natural movement.

This book is your comprehensive guide to face workouts. We'll delve into the science behind facial aging, explain how these exercises work, and provide a variety of targeted routines suitable for all skill levels. So, embark on this journey of natural rejuvenation and discover how a few simple exercises can unveil your most radiant and youthful self.

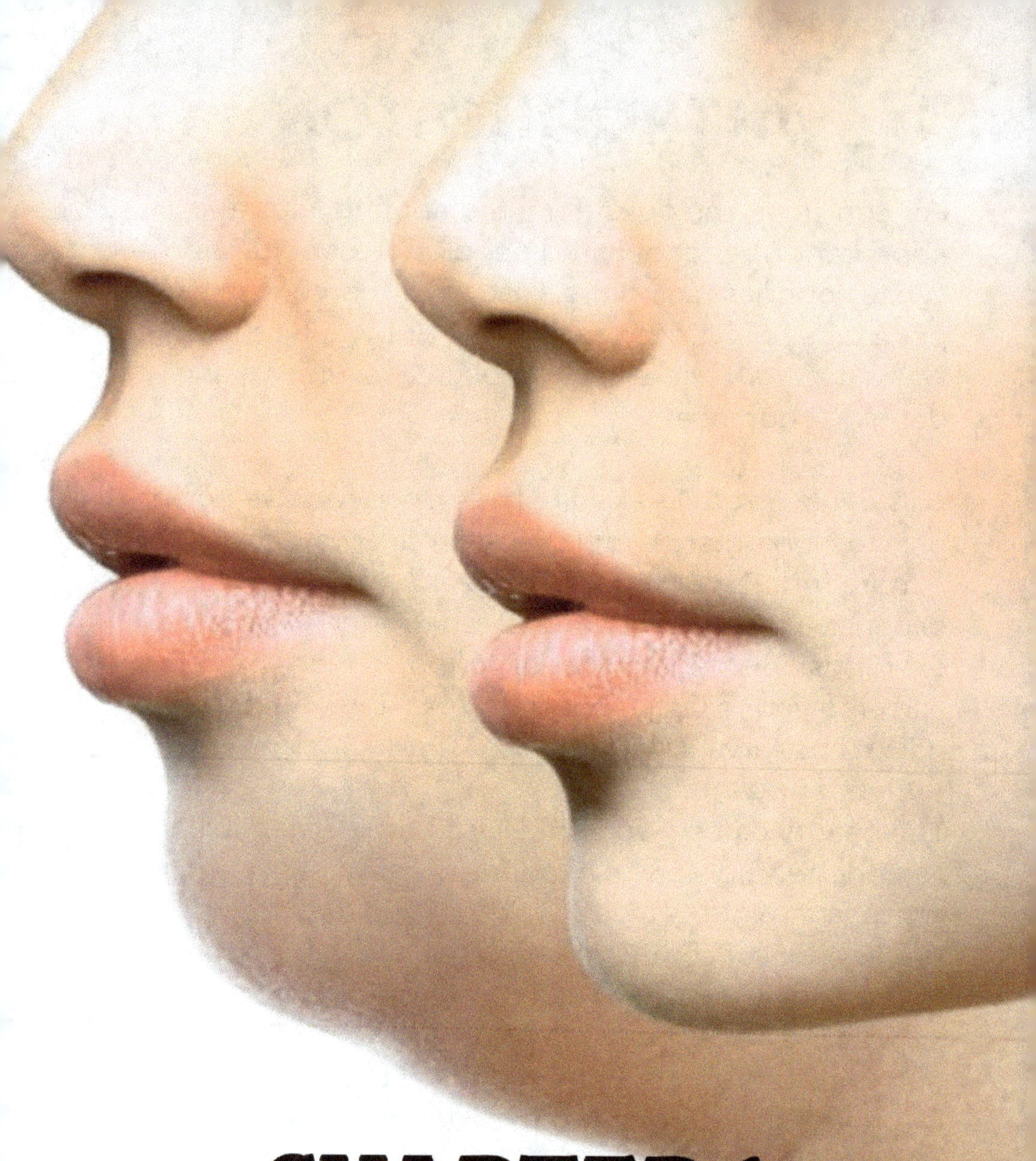

CHAPTER 1
Getting Started

What is face workout?

"Face yoga is a description for exercises performed to tone and stretch facial muscles," explains Dr. Amy B. Lewis, a dermatologist and certified yoga instructor based in New York. A more holistic approach to face sculpting than fillers and injectables, "face yoga has become extremely popular among existing yogis and newcomers," she says. Annelise Hagen, the author of The Yoga Face, is a certified yoga therapist who's been teaching and studying face yoga since 2005 (and traditional yoga since the early '90s). "Muscles lose mass and volume with age, so target-exercising face muscles as one would the body will sculpt, firm, and plump," Hagen says, noting that anyone can practice its methods "with caution and, hopefully, supervision" in the same way they would traditional workouts. "An older person can still drive benefit from practicing yoga techniques that promote facial rejuvenation, and a younger person can cultivate habits that will last a lifetime - plus prevent sags that could happen with atrophy and lack of exercise."

How Face Yoga Works

Face yoga is a gentle form of strength training for your face and neck that typically concentrates on one of the 57 facial muscles (or groups of muscles) at a time. "The more you repeat certain face yoga exercises, the more you may notice that the muscles and skin start to tighten," Lewis says. She mentions three main ways that face yoga may work for you: First, by stimulating muscles to improve their tone and tightness. Next, by increasing circulation and blood flow, "which helps skin heal and appear healthier," and finally, by reducing strain and tension in facial muscles "that are being contracted constantly during stress."

And while there are myriad versions to try, "the key to all of them is not to scrunch your face or squint a lot while doing these exercises," Lewis says. "The focus should be on lifting and expanding instead." She suggests practicing for at least 20 minutes a day for six weeks to see the benefits.

The Benefits of Face Yoga

The world is abuzz with the amazing benefits that come from practicing face yoga. Practicing face yoga is a natural way to maintain the toning of your facial muscles, keeping them looking young.

Toning Down Wrinkles

One standout benefit you'll love about face yoga exercises? They help reduce wrinkles. As our skin ages, it can become less elastic and cause wrinkles to form. But here's the good news: regular practice of these exercises strengthens your facial muscles, which results in smoother skin over time – say goodbye to those pesky crow's feet.

Brighter Skin Tone

Apart from fighting off wrinkles, another cool perk is improved skin tone. When done right (and trust me, consistency matters), these workouts stimulate blood circulation throughout your entire face, giving you a more even complexion that radiates healthiness.

Promoting Relaxation

You know what else makes this form of exercise so awesome? Just like traditional yoga techniques, focusing on each movement lets you connect mindfully with yourself, promoting relaxation – pretty handy considering how much tension we often hold within our faces without realizing.

- *Naturally Youthful Appearance:*

If there was ever a natural fountain-of-youth solution for maintaining younger-looking features, then this would be it. No need for invasive procedures or costly creams; just dedicated daily sessions can lead towards preserving youthfulness naturally through targeted movements designed specifically for every unique contour on your beautiful mug.

- *Increase Circulation:*

Last but certainly not least: one major appeal for many practitioners is that it's all-natural. Enhanced circulation ensures better oxygen supply, leading to healthier cells and ultimately resulting in glowing skin. So whether you're already studying face yoga or thinking about starting soon, remember â€" when practiced consistently alongside other forms such as Pilates â€" these routines offer countless ways towards achieving overall wellness while reducing signs of aging at the same time.

Tips for doing face yoga

Just like traditional yoga or Pilates, face yoga requires a strategic approach to reap the most benefits. Here are some useful tips that can enhance your facial fitness designed with face exercises and boost their effectiveness.
Start Slowly and Gradually Increase Intensity
The initial phase of practicing face yoga involves starting slow with gentle movements. It is essential to not push your facial muscles too hard, as this could cause harm. Instead, focus on performing each movement smoothly while gradually increasing intensity over time.

Mirror Usage is Key

A mirror becomes an essential tool when doing these target-exercising face muscle routines. By observing yourself perform each pose in front of a mirror, you ensure proper form and prevent unnecessary strain on those delicate muscles involved in creating our expressive facial expressions.

Frequent Practice Equals Better Results

Consistency is key when it comes to face yoga. Aim to have regular face yoga sessions in order to sustain the suppleness and strength of your facial muscles. Aim for regular sessions to maintain the tone and elasticity of your facial muscles.

Common mistakes in face yoga

If you're just beginning with face yoga, it's quite probable that some errors will be made. But don't worry. We've got your back.

Here are the most common errors and how you can avoid them while practicing face yoga exercises.

Mistake 1: Skimping on Pressure

You might think that being gentle is better when doing facial exercises – but hold up. That's where many folks trip up. Sure, we don't want any pain or discomfort during our routine, but applying just enough pressure is key for these techniques to work their magic on your facial muscles.

- To get this right, aim for a balance between force and comfort – feeling the stretch without straining.
- This will ensure effective improvement in lower cheek fullness as well as other benefits of practicing face yoga.

Mistake 2: Forgetting About Breathing

Breathing isn't just about keeping us alive – it plays an essential role in all forms of exercise, including facial fitness designed through face yoga.

1. A couple tips:
2. Incorporate deep inhales with each movement; exhale fully upon release.
3. The correct breathing technique helps skin heal by oxygenating cells while also promoting relaxation – a double win.

Mistake 3: Keeping Facial Muscles Tense Between Sets

- Failing to relax those hardworking muscles after each set? Big no-no.
- Why? Because rest periods allow muscle recovery – a crucial part of every workout regimen.
- Letting go of tension post-set prepares your target-exercising-face-muscles for another round so they can continue working towards achieving that healthy glow from within.
- Just like traditional body workouts need breaks, so does practicing these above-the-neck sculpting techniques.
- So remember – breathe out, let go, and give those stretched-out muscles some

How often do you need to practice face yoga to see results?

"Ideally every single day, if you want to see good results," says Hayashi. Wizemann agrees that consistency is the only key to success: "If you like a challenge and can stick to a 30-minute daily beauty routine for at least five months, you could possibly look a couple of years younger." But Wizemann adds that these exercises shouldn't replace the proven efficacy of anti-aging skin care and sun protection.

What face tools should you be using ?

There are so many beauty tools available now that it can be hard to know what will work for you.

As a Face Yoga practitioner and expert for the last 17 years, I believe that our hands are some of the best tools we can use. Using only your hands in a Face Yoga routine can exercise, massage, relax the face and even apply acupressure.

If you want to add a little variation to your routine, re-motivate yourself or work your skin in a different way, I have put together a list for you of some of my favourite face tools for you. They all can be used to complement the work you're already doing with your daily Facial Yoga and leave your skin looking and feeling glowing.

1. JADE ROLLER

A jade roller is great to use anytime in the day but I particularly recommend this crystal in the evenings as part of your bedtime routine.

Use the roller on a clean face with a few drops of the Fusion by Danielle Collins Pro Lift Facial Moisturising Serum, for the best results.

Jade has so many benefits for your face and is often known as the 'master crystal' for the skin. It is perfect for skin lifting and smoothing, it helps to boost the circulation in your face and is renowned for balancing the yin and yang in the body to maintain one's health.

Generally it's a good crystal for most people to use and particularly nice if you are looking for natural 'anti ageing' benefits.

A little tip...make sure you buy a jade roller that is really good quality. Some products say they are jade rollers when in fact they are made of glass or marble. If they aren't made of jade, you won't get all the goodness from the crystals!

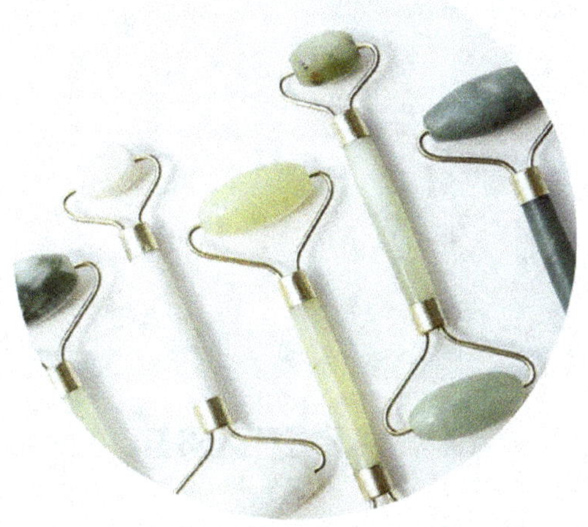

2. ROSE QUARTZ ROLLER

Rose quartz is a renowned crystal to use in the morning, In Traditional Chinese Medicine it is recommended to be used between early morning and 1pm.

The rose quartz roller is especially good if you have sensitive skin or skin that is inflamed and prone to blemishes. It will calm down inflamed and angry skin but take care not to use it on any areas of active acne, rosacea or eczema. It is also great for you if you are a teenager, have mature skin or often feel quite sensitive in your mind and body.

It is also very good if you suffer from puffy eyes, dark circles or dull skin in the morning. Make sure you keep this roller in the fridge so it's cold and refreshing when you use it on your skin. This will feel amazing when you use it under your eyes as it will help to leave them looking refreshed and de-puff them.

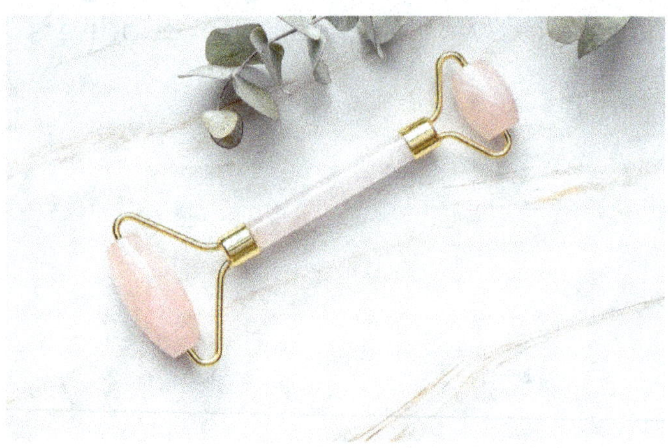

3. JADE GUA SHA

I love this product! The benefits of the Jade Gua Sha are almost endless.

Again…keep this one in the fridge for when you're ready to use it.

You can use this in so many ways. You can press and hold it on your skin when you wake up and it will help you with any under-eye puffiness. As well as reducing puffiness, it will also help with dark circles, lifting and firming the skin. Use the Gua Sha on acupressure points to help with any tension that is causing you headaches.

This Jade Gua Sha is beautiful quality, so you really get the full nourishing effect of the Jade.

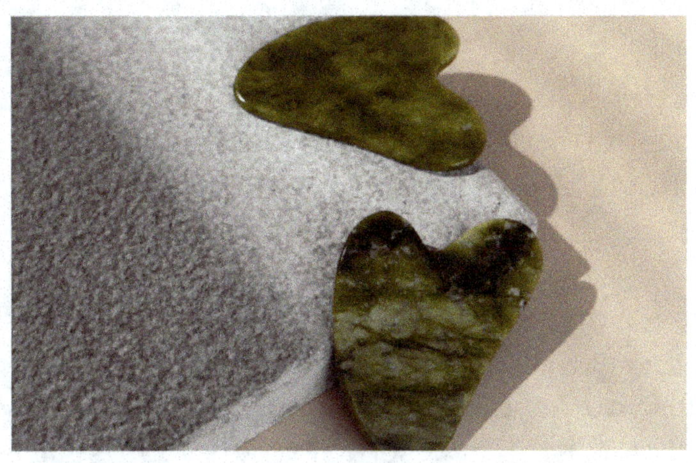

4. STAINLESS STEEL GUA SHA

Body Gua Sha is one of the most traditional and beneficial ways of using Gua sha because of it's ability to ease stress in the body and mind.

The Stainless Steel Gua Sha is perfect for using on your chest area, neck, lower back and shoulders. When we reduce strain from these areas we not only feel more comfortable but we indirectly help the face too. Less stress in the body always equals less lines on the face.

When you use the Stainless Steel Gua Sha, you might notice some redness but there shouldn't be any pain. The redness is good as it shows it's getting your blood circulating.

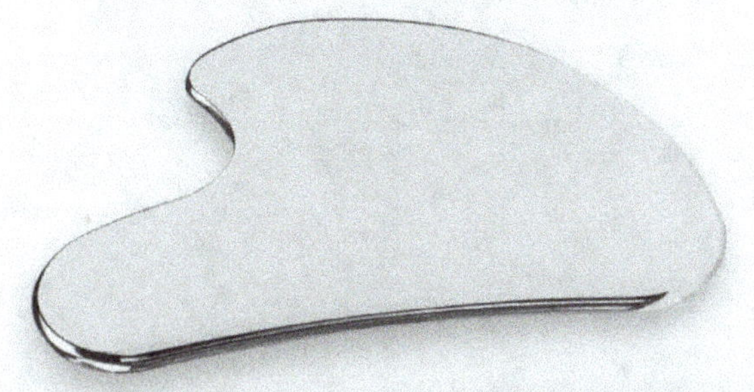

5. KANSA WAND

I love this Kansa Wand you can buy from Mauli Rituals.
It is a little bit more expensive than some other brands you can buy but it is beautifully made and such a useful tool to have.

The Kansa Wand is so good for massaging your skin and working on Ayuvedic 'Marma' or acupressure points.
Make sure you have clean skin and use lots of my Fusion By Danielle Moisturizing serum when you use it as, when you use the Wand it brings out a lot of acidity in the skin which can leave it looking a bit grey if you use no oil or have make up on.

This tool honestly feels SO good! It will lift and smooth your skin while leaving you relaxed in the process. Win win!

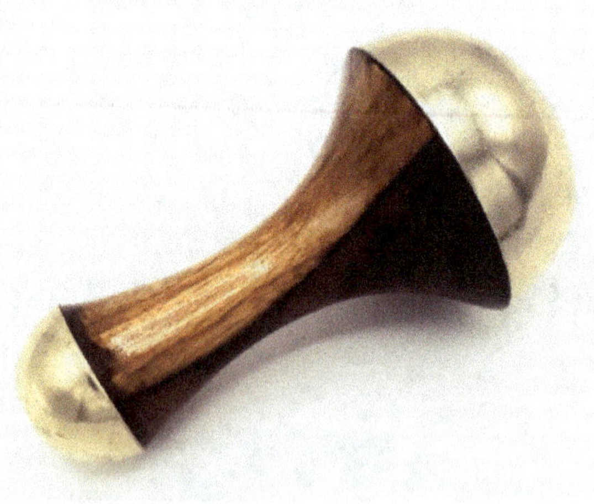

How to Do Face Yoga

- "There are so many different face yoga routines that you can do at home," says Serrador. "My favorite [routine] only has four steps." Before following a face yoga routine, you'll want to prep your skin. Start by cleansing your skin with your favorite face wash. (Right now, we're loving the CeraVe Hydrating Foaming Oil Cleanser.)
- Next, apply a facial essence over your skin with clean fingers or a cotton pad. For extra hydration, follow with a facial oil over your face and neck. As a last step, gently apply a moisturizer over your face and neck in an upward, circular motion.
- Once you've completed your skincare routine, it's time to start the yoga "poses." To do so, follow Serrador's instructions, below.
- **Step 1** Starting from the center of your chin, use a facial massager and roll it in light, upward strokes along the jawline towards your ear. Repeat on both sides of your face.
- **Step 2** Place the massager between your eyebrows — just above the nose — and roll upwards towards the hairline. Repeat this motion on the left and right sides of your forehead, too.
- **Step 3** Sweep the massager down your neck towards the collarbone. Repeat on both sides.
- **Step 4** Finally, starting at the top of your breastbone, massage outwards towards your lymph nodes. Repeat in each direction.

The Best Beginner Face Yoga Exercises

Don't have a facial massager or simply want some other face yoga poses to try? We've detailed a few simple face yoga exercises to include in your daily routine, below. The best part is that they'll only take a few minutes out of your day!

- **The Big O** This face yoga exercise, which Takatsu called "the big O," targets nearly all of the muscles in your face. Start by widening your eyes and making an "O" shape with your mouth by pressing your upper lip to your teeth. Basically, you'll be mimicking a surprised facial expression. Hold the pose for 10 seconds, then repeat.

- **Facial Lines** Facial lines are often formed from daily habits and expressions, whether that be smiling or furrowing your brow. This face yoga pose may help to offset some of those expressions we've all become accustomed to. Close your eyes and visualize the space between your eyebrows, allowing your face to relax. Then, form a very slight smile. Repeat as you wish.

- **Cheeks** Give your cheek muscles a workout by taking a deep breath and sucking in as much air as you can through your mouth. Puff the breath back and forth from cheek to cheek. After going back and forth a few times, release your breath.

- **Chin and Neck** Your neck is one of the most neglected areas of skin, which is why signs of aging can crop up prematurely here. Target this area by placing the tip of your tongue to the roof of your mouth and applying pressure. Point your chin towards the ceiling, then smile and swallow while pointing your chin at the ceiling.

- **Eyebrows** This face yoga pose isn't an instant eyebrow lift, but you may find benefits to completing it regularly. Place a finger under the center of each eye, pointing your fingers towards your nose. Open your mouth and curl your lips so that they hide your teeth, stretching your lower face. While still holding below your eyes, flutter the upper eyelids while looking at the ceiling.

- **Lips** Pucker up and blow a kiss! Press your lips into your hand, blow a kiss, and repeat to help give your lips the temporary appearance of more fullness.

- **Jawline Hooks** "Create a V-shape hook with your thumb and index finger and place [your hand] at the center of the chin with your thumb underneath," Theron explains. "Move the V along each side of the jawline, working slowly to contour and ease any tension." For this exercise, you'll want to apply medium pressure and repeat it eight times on each side.

- **V Eye Lifts** This is one of Theron's favorite massages for opening up the eyes. "Place two fingers on each side of the bridge of the nose up to the start of the eyebrow," says Theron. "Apply a little pressure and lift under the eyebrow, then split the fingers into a V-shape and let them glide out to the sides, still applying a little pressure. Repeat three times." For your under-eyes, use slightly less pressure so as not to drag the delicate skin in this area. "Place two fingers at the inner corner of the eye, split your fingers into a V-shape and let them glide out to the sides, finishing with a little lift and pressure at the temples. Repeat three times."

- **The Swan Neck** Another one of Takatsu's go-to exercises, the Swan Neck, helps tone your neck and jawline. Start by looking up and to the right at about a 45-degree angle, then pucker your lips towards the right. You should feel a stretch on the left side of your neck. After holding for five seconds, relax your muscles and return your gaze forward, then repeat the process on the other side. You can do this three times on each side. Don't forget to finish with a smile!

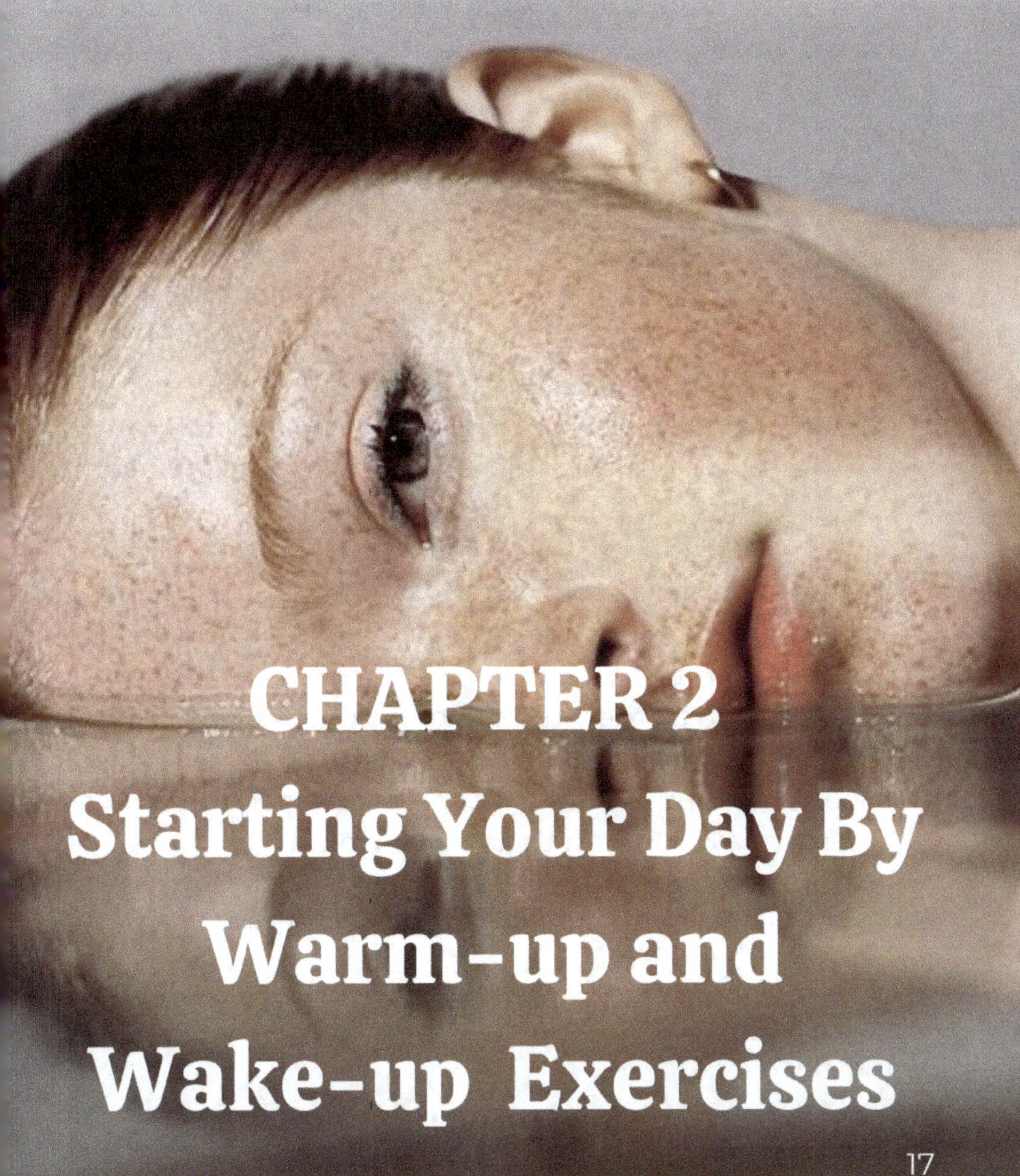

CHAPTER 2
Starting Your Day By
Warm-up and
Wake-up Exercises

Face Yoga Exercises for Morning

The best time to start your face yoga routine in the morning is after cleansing your face. You'll need a clean face and clean hands to do it. If your skin gets extra dry after cleansing you can put on some serum and start the exercises. The serum will moisturize, nourish and work as a lubricant while you warm up those sleepy muscles.We've combined a nice 5 steps routine for you to get a general impression of the morning face yoga. It starts with toning the biggest muscles first (neck and forehead) and works its way to the more delicate area (eyes) as you get a better grip on the process.

Exercise 1. Warm-Up

Every physical exercise routine starts with a warm-up. And face yoga is no different. This exercise will gently wake up your face and bring energy and warmth to your face.How to do it:

- Put your hands to your forehead, and very gently begin tapping it with your fingertips.
- Slowly begin to move from the forehead to the under-eye area and all the way to the neck.
- When you're done tapping through every cell of your face and neck, bring your hands together. Start energetically rubbing them to warm up.
- Put warm hands on your face.
- Breath in. Breath out. Feel stress and tension leave your facial muscles.
- Put your hands down. You are ready to start.

Exercise 2. Neck

The main goal of this exercise is to promote lymphatic drainage. This will reduce the morning face puffiness, and bring color and youth to your complexion. It also helps to wipe the pillow marks off your neck, if there are any.
How to do it:
- Put both your hands just below the ears and the jawline.
- Using all of your fingers to gently press the skin and move from the top of your neck towards the collar bone.
- Repeat for 30 seconds.

Exercise 3. Forehead

This exercise will massage and release the tension of the big muscle at the front of your forehead. Bye-bye, frown wrinkles! It also has the botox-like effect. The more you do this massage, the more relaxed your forehead will be during the day. No more over-raising or over-furrowing your brows. How to do it:
- Make hands into fists.
- Put them to the center of your forehead.
- Horizontally move fists from the center towards your hairlines.
- Repeat for 30 seconds. Or as long as you want.

Exercise 4. Cheeks

This exercise is an alternative to fillers. It helps to defeat gravity and firm up sagging skin. It also tones your cheek muscles, giving them a lift and a radiant skin glow.
How to do it:

- Fill up one of your cheeks with air.
- Pretend that you're using mouthwash and move the air from one cheek to another.
- Continue for 1 minute and relax.
- Repeat 5 to 10 times for best results.

Exercise 5. Eyes

This last massage seems simple, but it is the top choice when dealing with the puffy eyes and dark circles. Add your favorite eye product, try closing your eyes and fully relaxing while doing this exercise. How to do it:

- Use your index or ring finger to tap gently around your eye area in circles.
- Continue up to 1 minute

3 Things To Do After Your Morning Face Yoga Routine

- *Give yourself a credit*

You did it! You've carved out time for yourself, immersed into self-care and now you look fabulous. Your morning face is not a morning face anymore.

- *Continue with your morning skincare*

Your face is now prepped to make the best of the skincare ingredients. Don't forget to apply your moisturizer and other beauty products, and top it up with at least 30SPF sunscreen for best protection.

- *Drink water*

Your face just had a workout! Drink up and help your tissues and skin to stay hydrated.

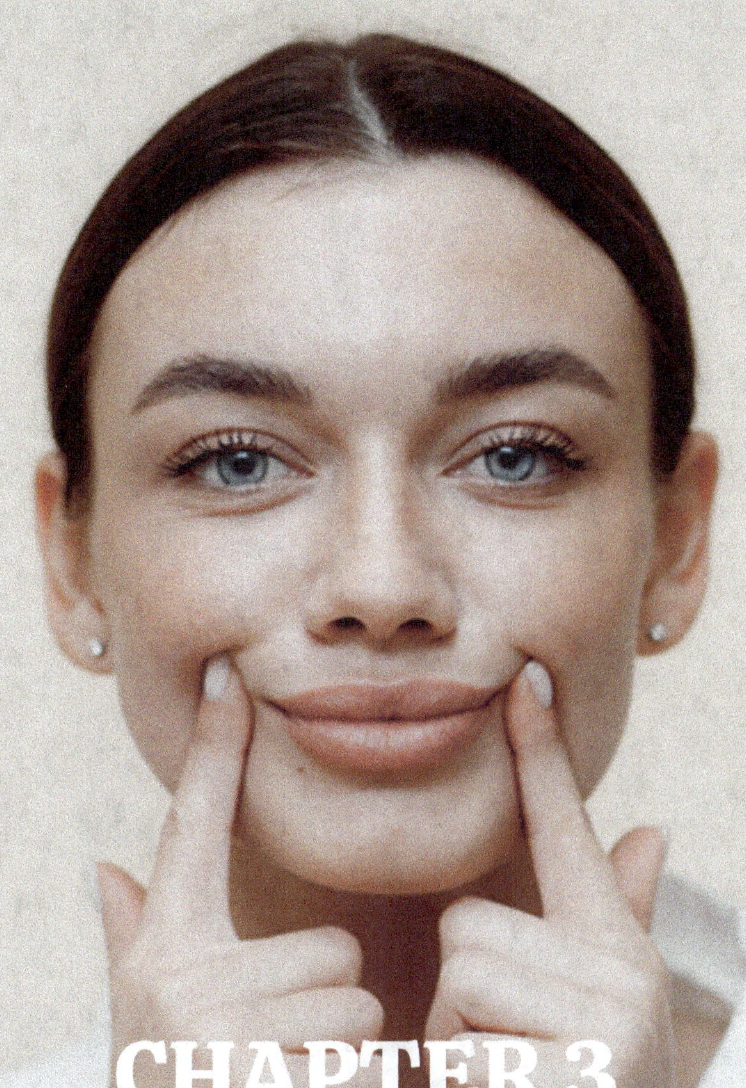

CHAPTER 3
Fundamental Face Workout

Types of Facial Exercises

Here are a few facial exercises that one can practice to keep your facial skin looking healthy and fresh.

A) Brow Raiser:

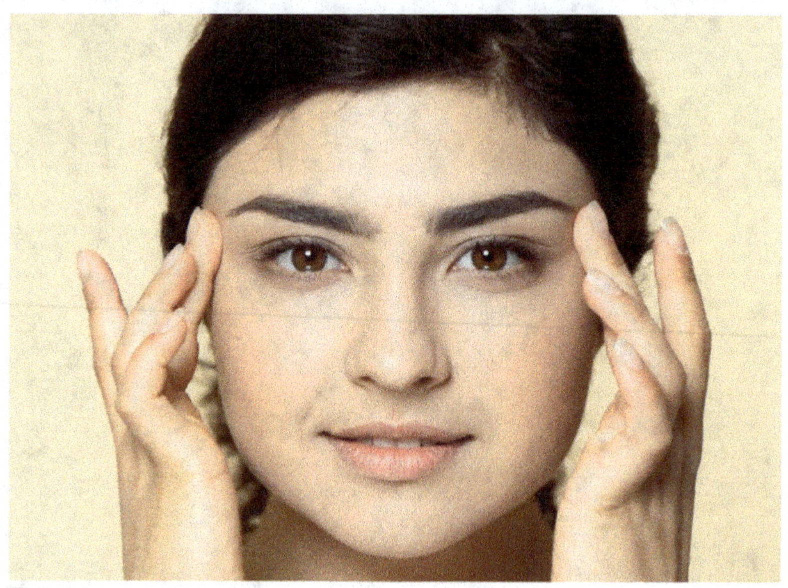

- Make a closed peace sign with your index and middle fingers
- Gently press the skin down with your fingertips across your brows
- Raise and drop your brows while using the weight of your fingernails to provide resistance
- Count to ten
- Finish six sets of this exercise everyday

B) Forehead smoother:

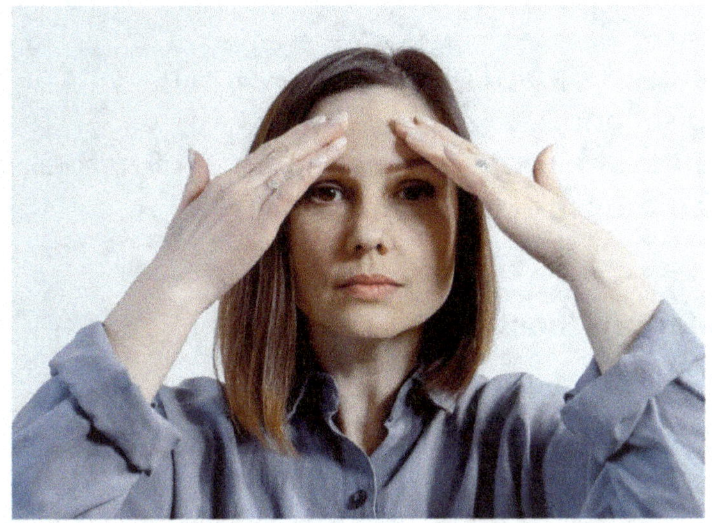

- How to do: Place both hands on your forehead and gently sweep them outward, applying slight pressure.
- Technique: Use smooth, controlled motions to avoid unnecessary friction.
- Benefits: Reduces forehead lines and wrinkles, promoting a smoother complexion.

C) Nasolabial Line Smoother:

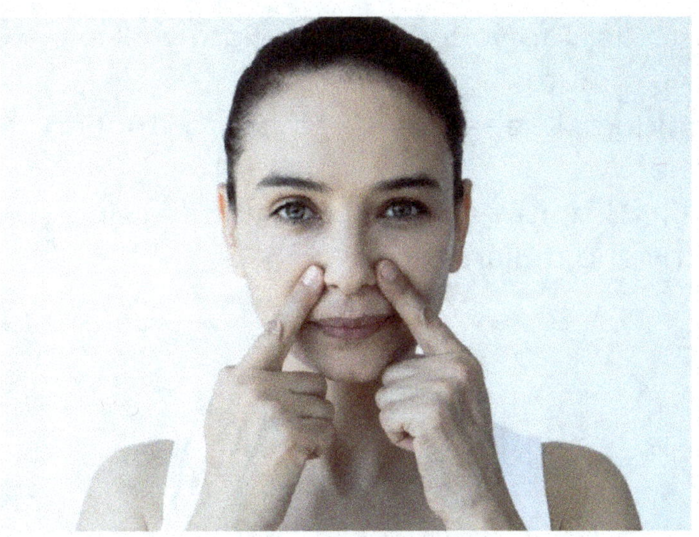

- How to do: Smile widely, then use your fingers to smooth out the lines that form around your nose and mouth.
- Technique: Apply light pressure, and repeat the motion for 30 seconds.
- Benefits: Minimizes the appearance of nasolabial lines, promoting a more youthful smile.

D) Circulation Booster:

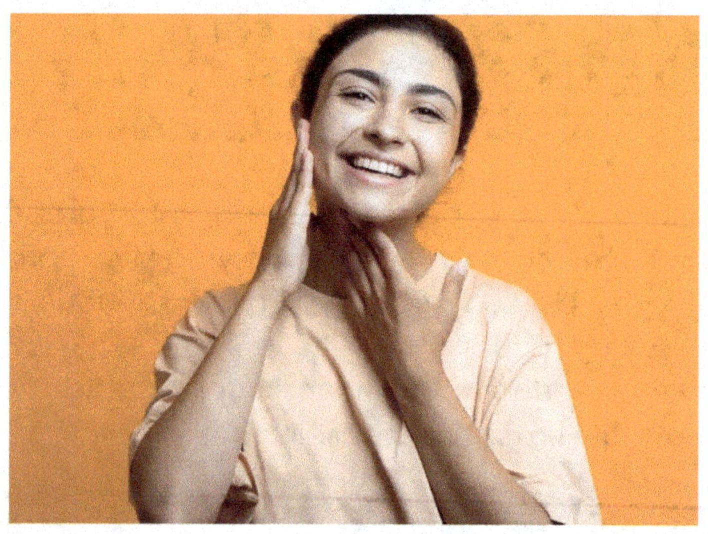

- How to do: Tap your fingertips lightly all over your face for one minute.
- Technique: Use a gentle tapping motion to avoid irritation.
- Benefits: Improves blood circulation, giving your skin a healthy and radiant glow.

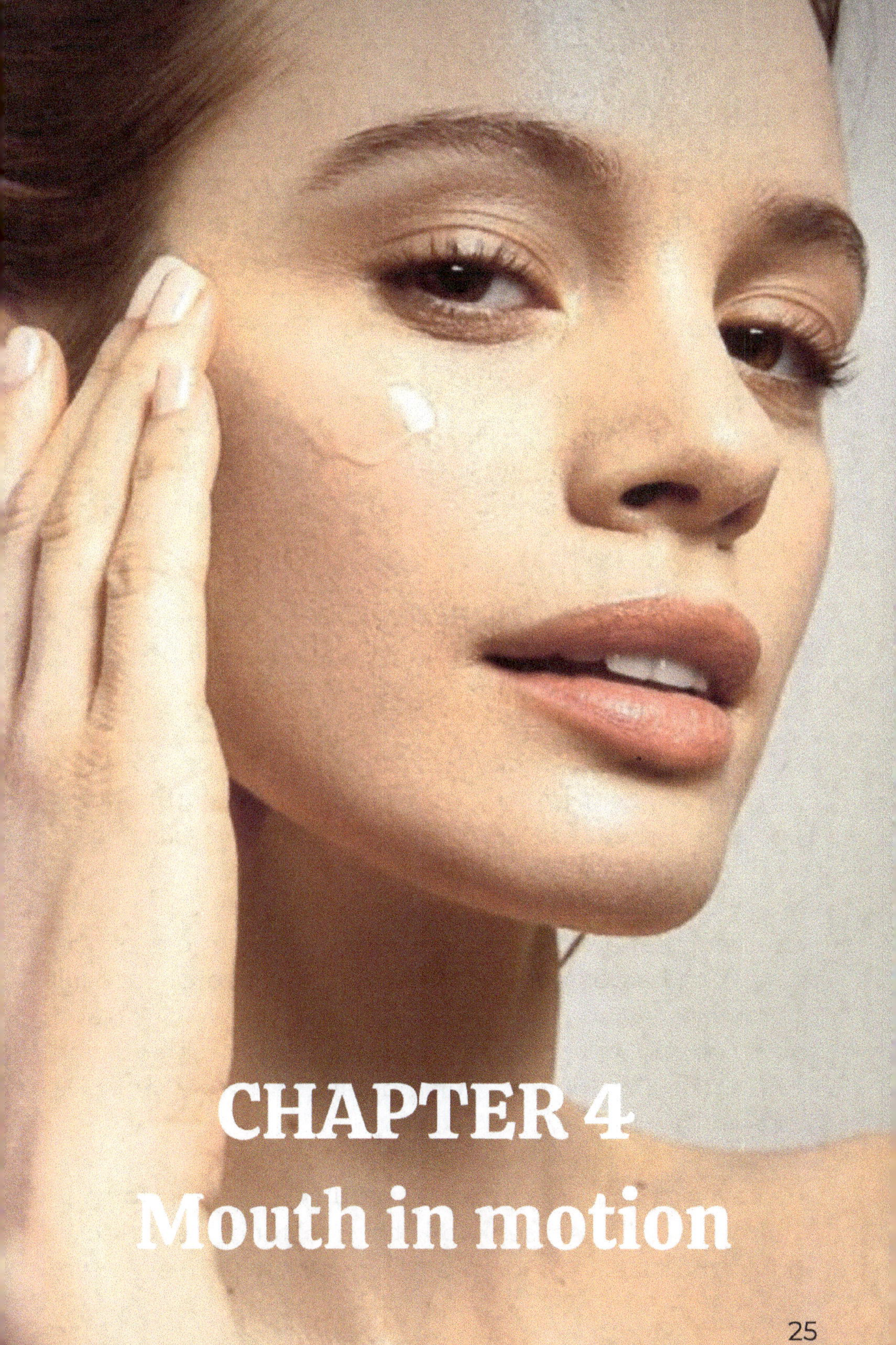
CHAPTER 4
Mouth in motion

Lift your mouth corners naturally

As we get older our muscles naturally start to lose strength. This includes the muscles in our faces. One of the side effects of this is that the corners of our mouths can start to drop down, making us look like we're unhappy, even when we're feeling perfectly happy and content.

We may also notice drooping in our cheeks, or a slight asymmetry in the different sides of our faces. So, in this post, I'm going to show you three facial exercises that target these areas and help to lift the mouth corners naturally.

These three techniques are quick and simple to do. In total, the full routine should only take a few minutes, so it is hopefully easy to fit it into your day.

You might decide to do these exercises as part of your morning or evening skincare routine (or both). Many people find it easiest to remember to do the exercises if they integrate them into their existing habits.

However, the beauty of face yoga is that most of the moves can be done anywhere. You don't need any special equipment – just your hands and perhaps a mirror and some serum. So, you could easily do these techniques in front of the TV, during a quick break from work, or while you're in the shower.

The key is to do the techniques regularly. Like any form of exercise, facial exercises work best to tone the muscles and lift the face if you do them consistently – ideally every day.

GET SET UP

Make sure your hands are clean before starting any face yoga sequence. Ideally, you want a clean face too, which is why many people like to do this as part of their skincare routine before they apply makeup.

This sequence only requires a minimal amount of touch, however, so you can get away with doing it during the day too.

Find a comfortable spot to sit or stand. It helps to have a mirror to hand for some of these exercises, so you can make sure you are maintaining symmetry as you hold the poses.

If you have some serum to hand, apply a few drops to the skin around your mouth and lower cheeks. I like to use my Fusion by Danielle Collins Pro Lift Facial Moisturising Serum, which is lovely for face yoga.

Take a few deep, calming breaths through your nose. And you are ready to start.

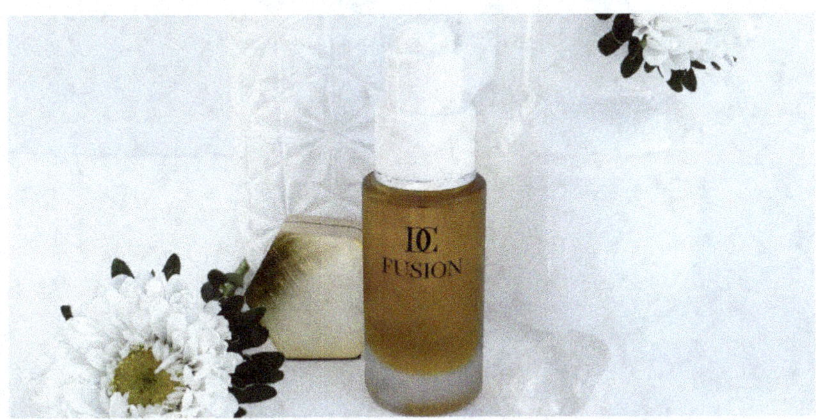

1. LIP TUCK

Tuck your lips in, keeping your mouth closed, and activate your muscles to turn the corners of your mouth up.

Check in the mirror to see if any lines are forming around your mouth. Use your index fingers to gently smooth any lines that do appear away. Keep your fingers on either side of your mouth so that your skin stays smooth while you hold the pose. We never want to create any fresh lines while doing face yoga!

Hold here for about 20 seconds. You'll feel your muscles working. This exercise helps to tone and lift the muscles around your mouth, tightening and tautening the attached skin and helping to lift the corners of your mouth.

Release for a few breaths and then repeat this exercise three more times.

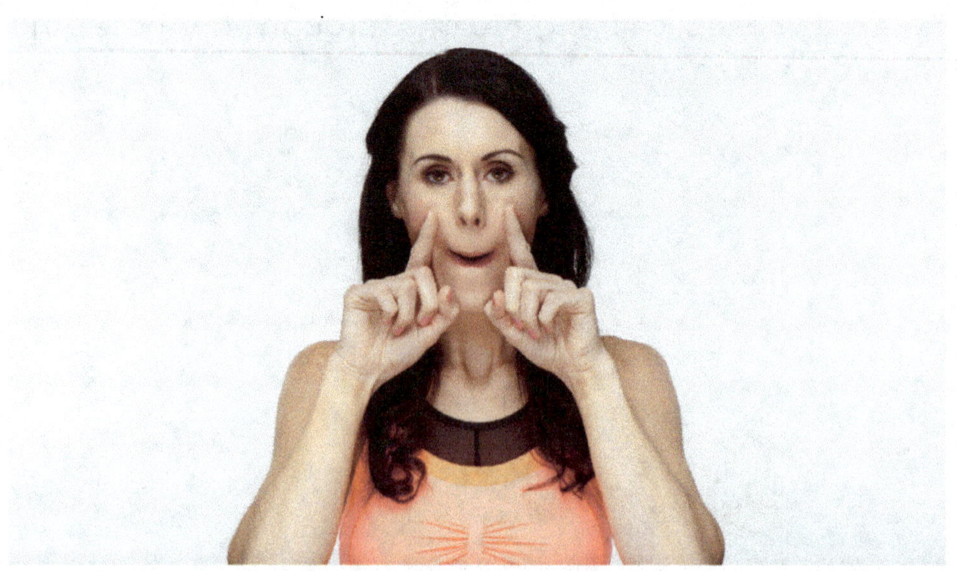

2. SMILE

Relax the muscles around your mouth and then lightly smile, keeping your lips together.

Place your index fingers on the corners of your mouth. Hold here, breathing deeply in and out through your nose.

As well as helping to encourage your mouth into this upward position, this exercise gives a boost to the energy and circulation, making your lower face look fresher and brighter.

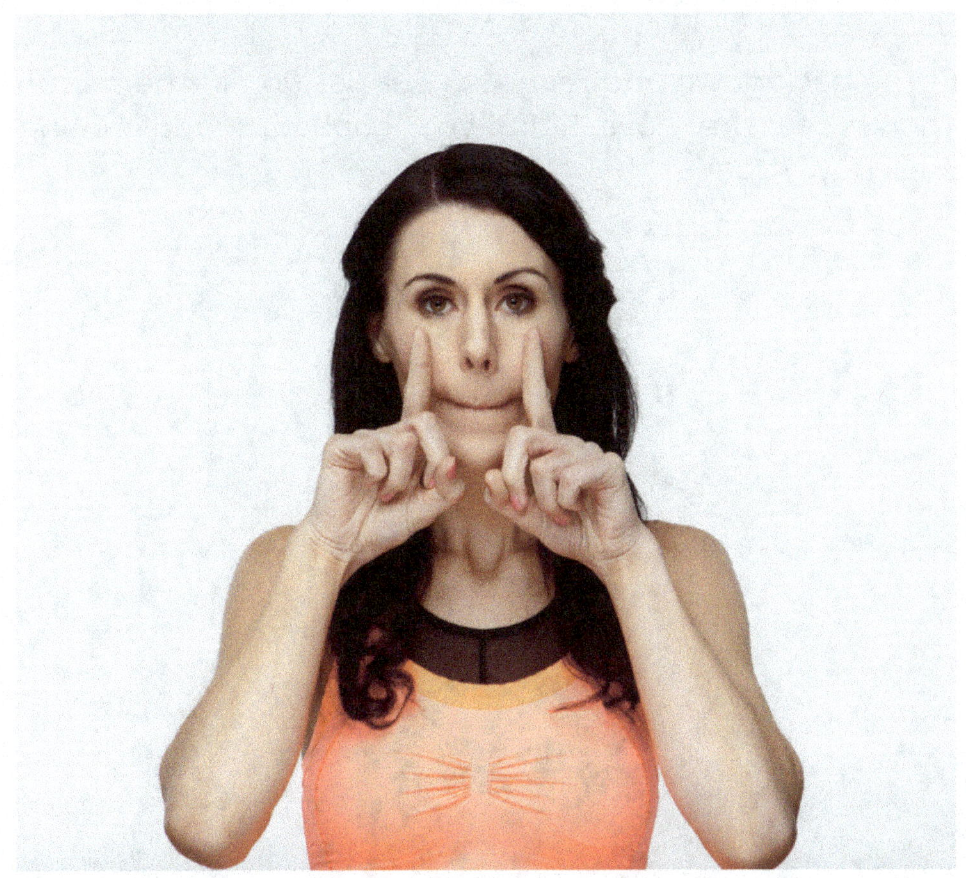

3. WRAP LIPS WITH HEAD TILT

Open your mouth a little so that you can wrap your lips around your teeth. Lift the corners of your mouth up as though you were smiling.

Once again, use your index fingers to smooth out any lines by placing them on either side of your mouth while you hold the pose. Use your mirror to make sure both sides of your mouth are symmetrical as you do this exercise.

Keeping your mouth and fingers in place, gently tilt your head back until you are looking up at the ceiling.

Come back down and recheck your position in the mirror. Then repeat the move, tilting your head back and coming back down again.

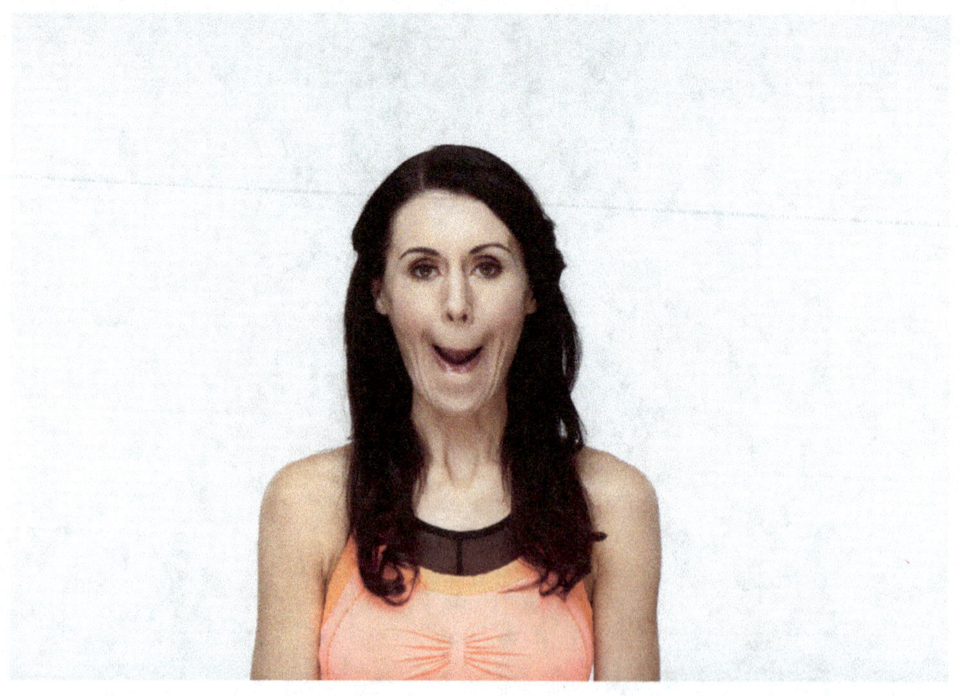

FINISH

Bring your hands back down and release your lips. Take a few deep breaths to finish, focusing on relaxing and releasing tension from the muscles of the lower face.

Hopefully, the muscles around your mouth feel like they've had a good workout. Over time, as you continue to do these exercises regularly, you'll begin to see an improvement in the symmetry of this area. You should also notice that the corners of your mouth naturally come into a more smiling, upward position.

I love to share simple, quick, but effective tips like these with all of you.

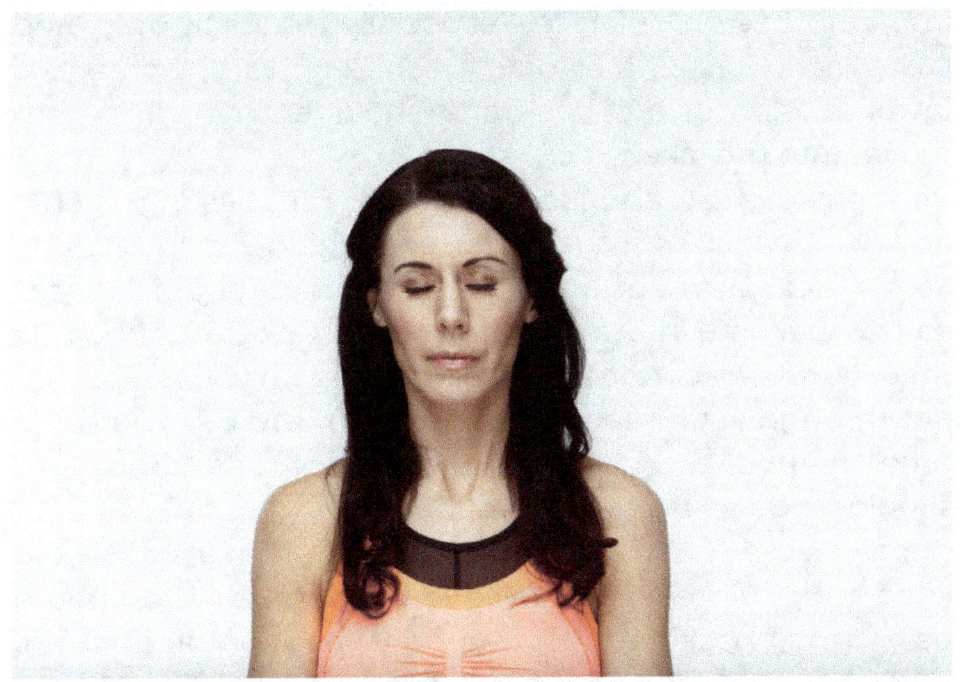

Facial massages for reducing JOWLS

I'm going to walk you through three of my favourite massage techniques for lifting and sculpting the lower face.

These moves are designed to increase blood circulation and tone the muscles, reducing any sagging that is starting to appear in this area.

Before we get onto the massage techniques themselves though, I just wanted to mention the importance of posture. If you are a long-time follower this is something you'll have heard me talk about regularly, but I always think it is worth reiterating.

We tend to overlook the importance of posture and the impact it has on our faces, especially the neck, chin, and jaw. When we spend all day hunched forward, it creates a lot of tension in our back and shoulders, which in turn moves into the face.

Poor posture can also lead to weaker muscles in the chin and neck, which eventually causes sagging and loose skin.

So, as you go through this massage routine, I also want you to become more mindful of your posture. Imagine that you have a cord running all the way up your spine and out through your head, pulling you upwards. At the same time, ground down through your feet and drop your shoulders down away from your ears.

Good posture naturally helps your lower face look more lifted and sculpted. Whenever you remember through the day, come back into this upright position and it will gradually start to feel more familiar and be easier to maintain.

With that in mind, let's look at these massage techniques for reducing jowls.

Lift your mouth corners naturally 2

BEFORE YOU START

The key to any facial massage is to make sure you have clean hands, a clean face, and have applied some serum to give your skin a lovely glide. I always use the Fusion by Danielle Collins Pro Lift Moisturising Serum.

Take a few long, slow breaths in and out through your nose to help yourself feel relaxed and centred before you begin the massage.

Then, you are ready to start.

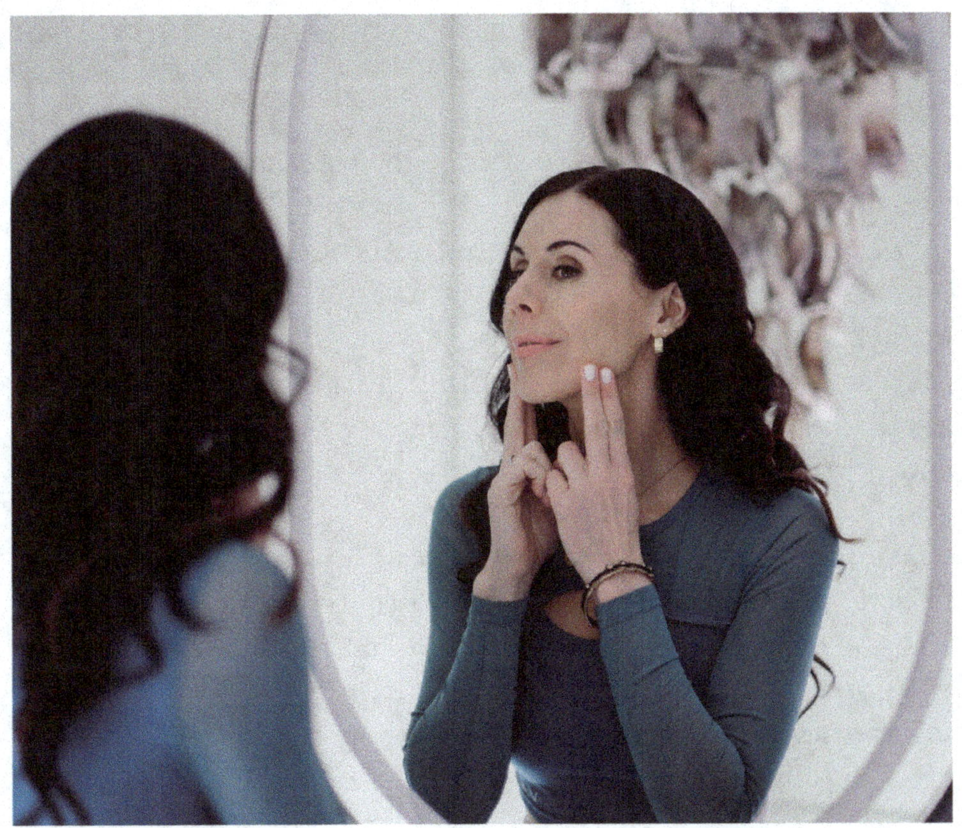

1. JAW MASSAGE

Take your index and middle fingers on both hands and place them to either side of your chin.

Keeping your fingers in contact with your skin, use a circular motion to slowly massage along your jawline, working out from your chin towards your ears.

Once you reach the area behind your earlobes, lift your fingers off and bring them back to your chin to start the massage again.

Next, use your thumbs to stroke along the underside of your jawbone. Again, you want to work outwards from your chin and lift off once you reach your ears.

Then, form a V-shape with your index and middle fingers. Alternating sides, smooth along your jawline from your chin to your ears.

All of these techniques are great for releasing tension and boosting blood circulation. By working outwards and upwards, we encourage that natural muscle lifting.

Facial massage also helps to stimulate the flow of energy – known as prana in yoga or Qi in Traditional Chinese Medicine. If that energy is very stagnant or blocked in a particular area, it can show up as wrinkles, dullness, or sagging skin.

With face yoga, we're always aiming to address issues holistically. Yes, we want to stimulate blood circulation, release muscle tension, and lift the face. But we also want to work on an energetic level to unblock any stagnant areas and get everything flowing freely again.

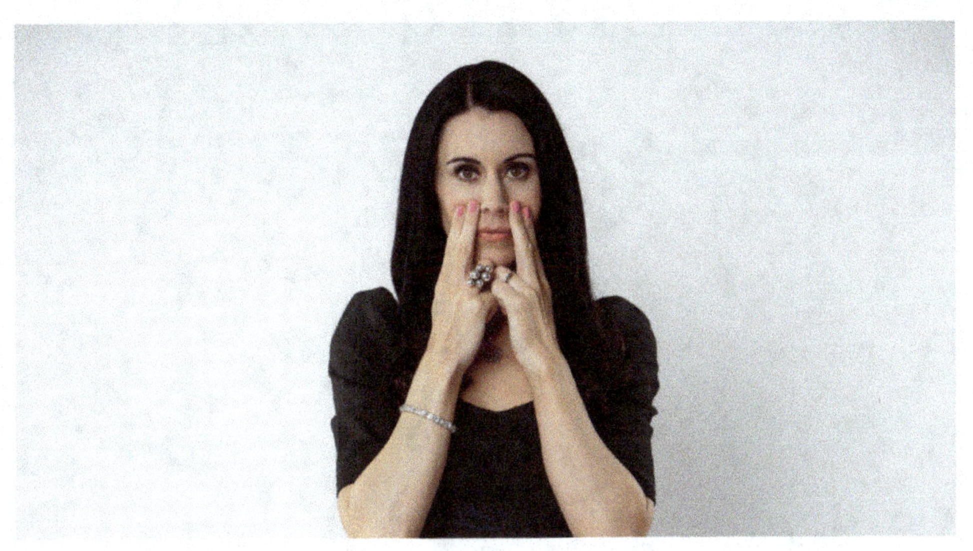

2. NASOLABIAL FOLDS

Next, we're moving to focus on the area around the mouth and nose. Many of us find lines developing here or notice the skin starting to sag as we get older. And sagging here can obviously contribute to the appearance of jowls too.

Massaging this area helps again to boost blood circulation, bringing plenty of fresh nutrients and oxygen to the skin and muscles. Of course, it also releases any stagnant energy or blockages that have built up.

Take your middle and index fingers together and bring them to your jawbone, on either side of your chin. Using a circular motion, massage up past your mouth and to the outside of your nostrils, following the nasolabial folds (the lines that go from the corners of your mouth to your nose).

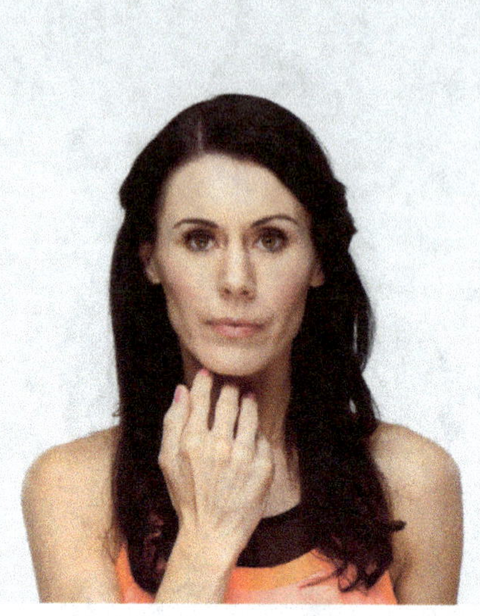

Once you get to your nose, lift off and return to your jaw to repeat the action again.

3. NECK

Finally, we're going to finish up by massaging the top part of the neck and under the chin.

Gently tilt your head back so that you can access the area more easily. Using both hands, stroke upwards over your neck and under your chin. You may need to apply some more serum if you didn't put any on your neck to start with.

Next, hold one hand under your chin, palm facing down. Use the tops of your fingers to tap upwards, massaging the skin under your chin.

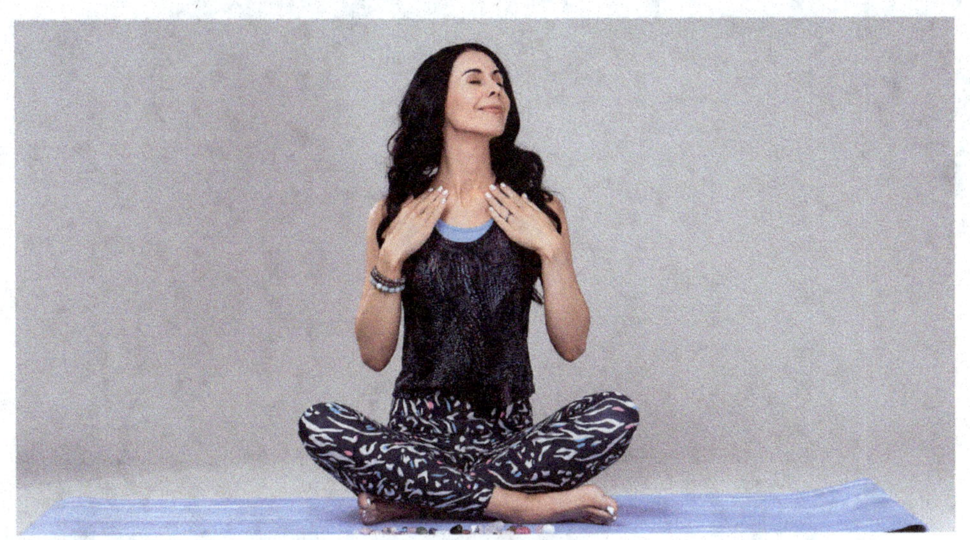

ALL DONE!

I said at the start about the importance of posture and how it connects to the face. Really, the thing you realise when you practice face yoga is that everything is connected.

The upper body is connected to the neck, chin, and jaw, the neck is connected to the lower face, the lower face is connected to the upper face. So, if you want to reduce the appearance of jowls, you don't just want to target that area but also the areas around it – such as the neck and the lower face.

That's why I've given you massage ideas for all three areas here, so you can address them together and really get the energy flowing everywhere.

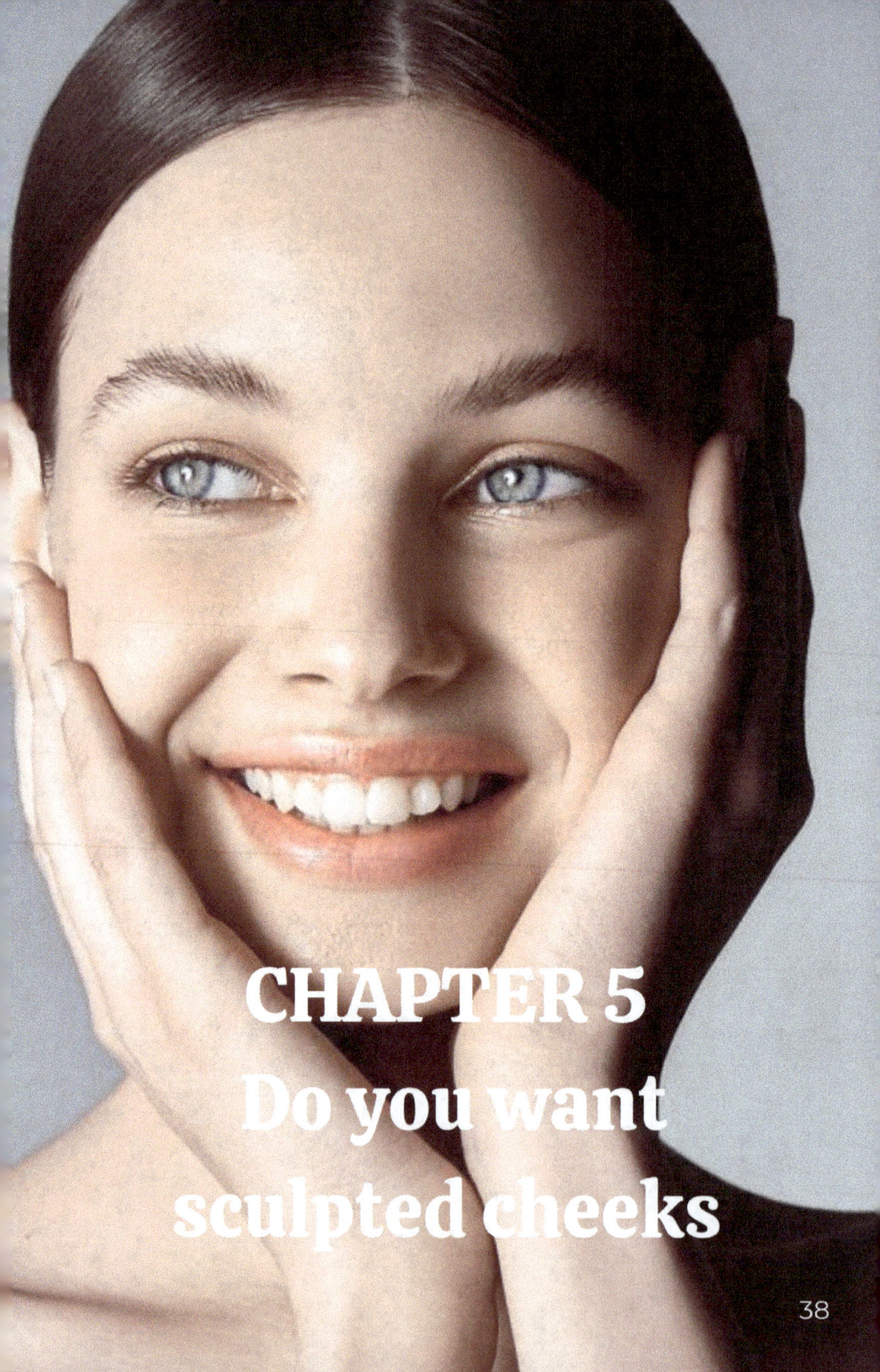
CHAPTER 5
Do you want
sculpted cheeks

Sculpt the cheekbones naturally with 5 facial exercises

I'm going to take you through a quick and easy Face Yoga sequence that focuses on defining and sculpting your cheekbones. You might even see the effects of some of these techniques instantly, so it is a great set of moves to use just before you go out.

Of course, we can't change our underlying bone structure, even with Face Yoga. But what we can do is sculpt and tone the muscles, release tension, and brighten the skin. This makes everything look more lifted and defined.

Plus, like any Face Yoga routine, this short sequence gives you a moment to focus on self-care. It helps you to feel better on the inside, which is ultimately what Face Yoga is all about.

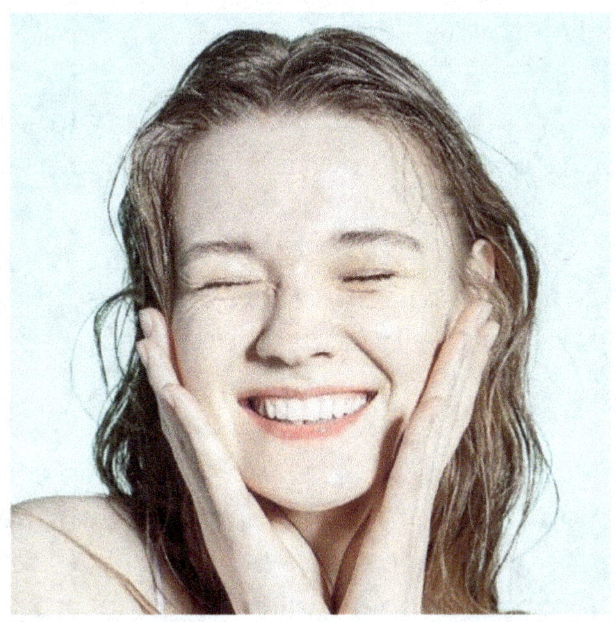

GETTING STARTED

Make sure you have clean hands and a clean face before you start this Face Yoga sequence. It's a quick routine and should only take five minutes, so it hopefully fits well into your existing skincare regime. If you are getting ready to go out, this is a great set of moves to do before you put your makeup on.

However, like any Face Yoga move, these techniques work best when you do them regularly.

Apply a few drops of the Fusion by Danielle Collins Facial Serum. This serum is specially formulated for use with Face Yoga and helps your fingers glide easily over your face. It is also packed with high-performing organic seed oils to nourish and moisturise your skin.

You can use the serum instead of your usual moisturiser or layer moisturiser over the top – no need to wash it off as it absorbs easily into the skin.

When you're ready, take a few deep, calming breaths through your nose. Feel your abdomen rise as you inhale and fall as you exhale.

As we work through this short Face Yoga sequence, try to keep that focus on the breath. Count to four as you inhale and then exhale for a count of six.

Finally, work to your own level with all these techniques. I encourage you to feel into your intuition and let it guide you – perhaps you feel that you want to spend a little longer with some of the moves or want to adjust the pressure to suit your own skin.

1. FLICK

Take your index and middle fingers under your cheekbones, starting close to your nose. Flick your fingers up and out as you work along beneath your cheekbones.

When you get to your ears, replace your fingers near your nose and repeat the move.

This releases tension and tightness in the cheek area. It also boosts blood circulation, giving you nourished and glowing skin.

The effects of this technique are almost instantaneous, making your cheekbones look more sculpted and defined straight away.

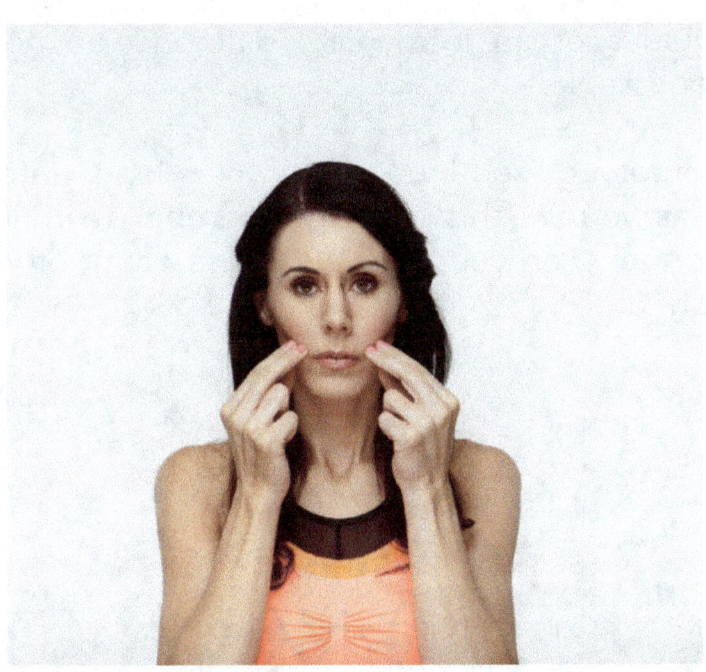

2. HOOKS

Form your index fingers into a hook shape. Using the middle knuckle, stroke beneath your cheekbones, working out from your nose.

Repeat the move for 30 seconds to a minute, lifting off when you reach your ears and starting again from your nose.

This beautifully calming move brings a warm tingle to the cheek area, which is a great indicator of increased blood circulation. All that fresh blood brings oxygen and nutrients to your skin cells, helping your skin look bright and glowing.

If you look in the mirror after working through this routine, you should spot an immediate difference in how your cheekbones look.

Don't forget to continue with your long, intentional breaths as you do this move. Remember to make your exhale longer than your inhale (in for a count of four, out for a count of six).

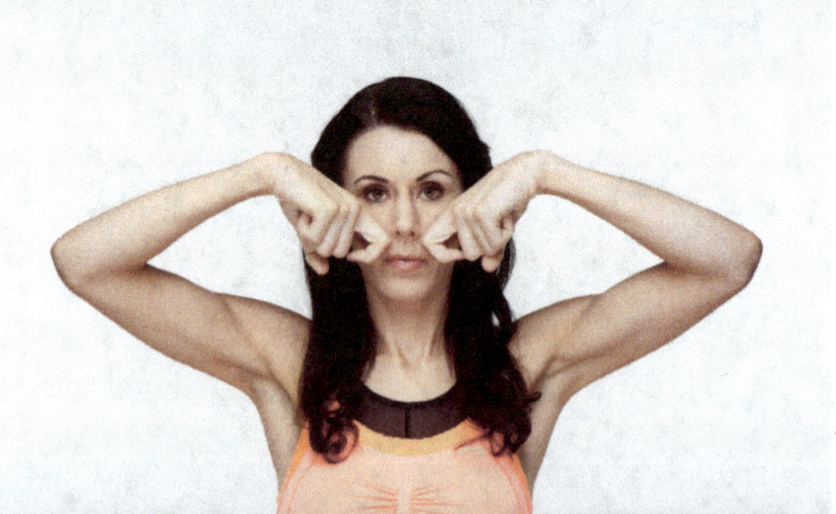

3. PINCH

Using two fingers and your thumb, pinch and release along your cheekbones.

The aim here is to pinch down into your muscles, not pull and drag the skin itself. Try to get your thumb right under your cheekbones to really lift and define them.

As you do this move, concentrate on relaxing the rest of your face and releasing any tightness. The jaw and forehead are two areas where many of us hold a lot of tension, especially when we're stressed or overwhelmed.

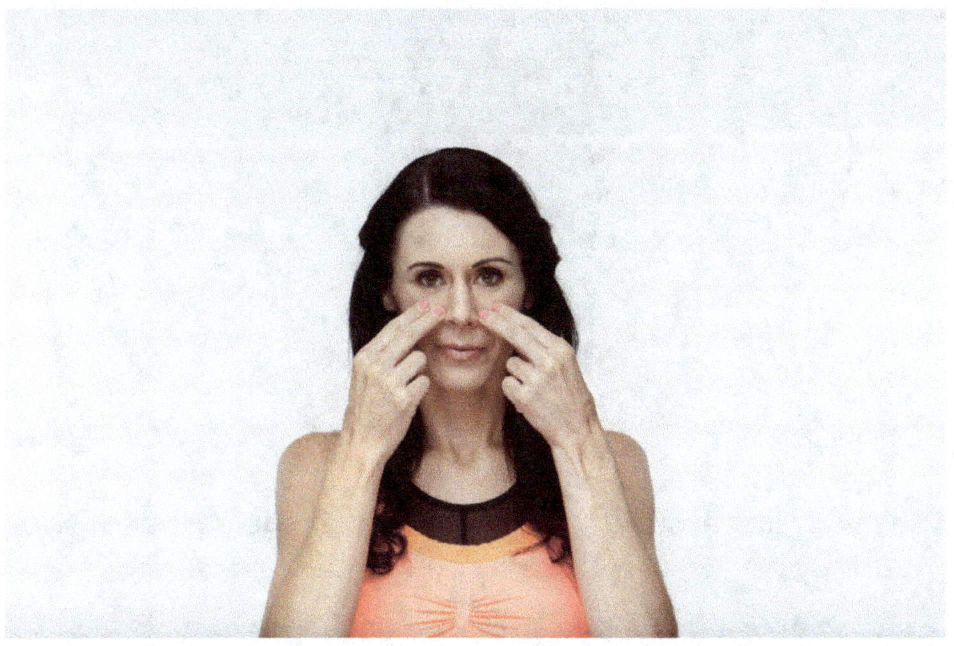

As you pinch, consciously work on relaxing these areas, releasing tension with every exhale.

4. MUSCLE STRENGTHENING

This facial exercise works to strengthen and tone the muscles in your cheeks, which in turn lifts and tightens the attached skin, giving you more defined cheekbones.

Like any form of exercise, this technique works best if you do it regularly. Every day, if possible.

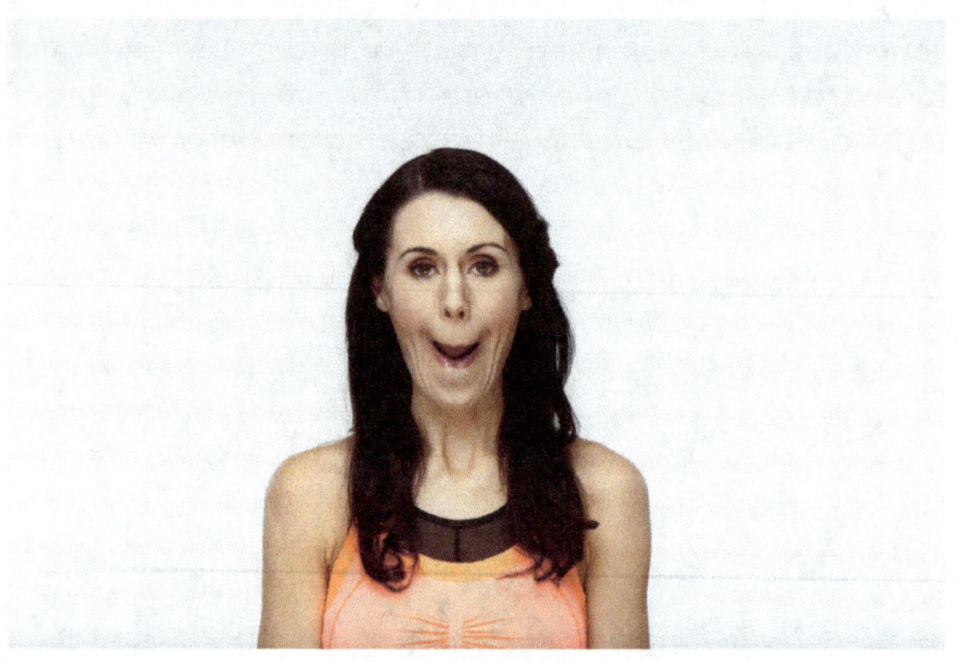

Tuck your lips around your teeth and lift the corner of your mouth up.

It is best to do this in front of a mirror. If you see any lines appearing around your mouth when you take this pose, use your index fingers to smooth out the skin.

Hold the pose for a count of 20. Release and then take it again.

5. TAP

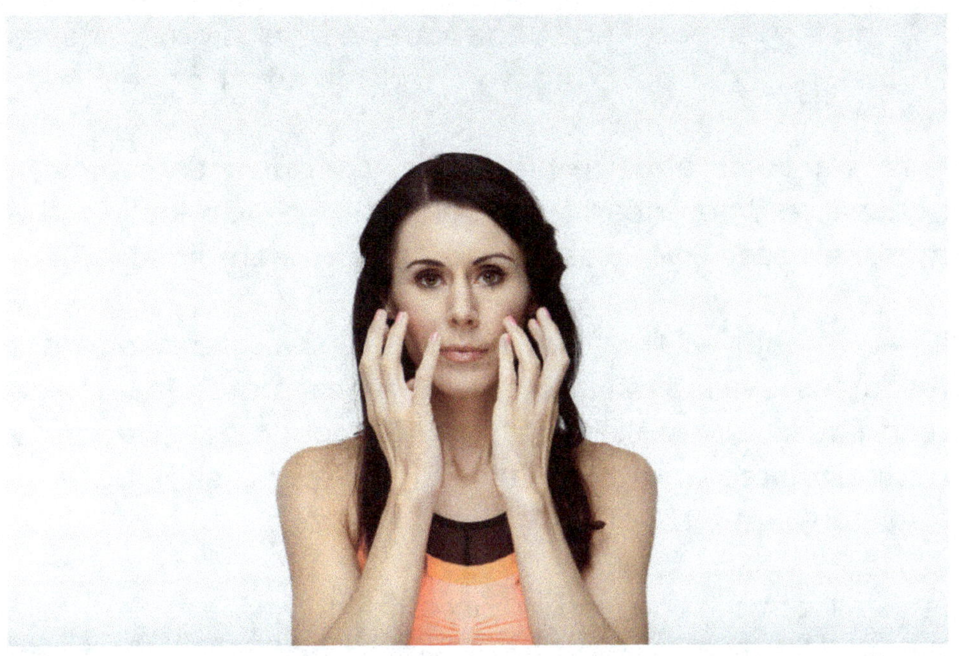

Using all your fingertips, tap rapidly over the whole cheek area for happy, tingly cheeks.

This simple technique is one of my favourites for boosting blood circulation, encouraging lymphatic drainage, and getting energy flowing. Plus, it feels wonderful and leaves you with skin that feels bright and awake.

As you tap, remember to focus on your breathing. Feel the tension leaving your face, especially your forehead and jaw. Concentrate on softening and releasing any tightness.

FINISHED!

Finish off this short Face Yoga routine by closing your eyes and taking a few deep breaths. And you are all done!

This is a quick and simple sequence, but it can make a noticeable difference to your cheekbones. Go look in the mirror and see if you can see an improvement already.

If you've enjoyed this focused class, I have plenty of other resources available to help you learn more Face Yoga techniques. Not only does regular Face Yoga give you a naturally lifted and toned face and glowing skin, but it is also a brilliant form of self-care.

I talk a lot about the importance of taking time for yourself. Modern life is pressured and busy, especially for women. We're often so busy taking care of others that we neglect our own needs. Putting aside a few minutes a day to concentrate on yourself and nourish your skin with your loving touch can do wonders for your mental wellbeing.

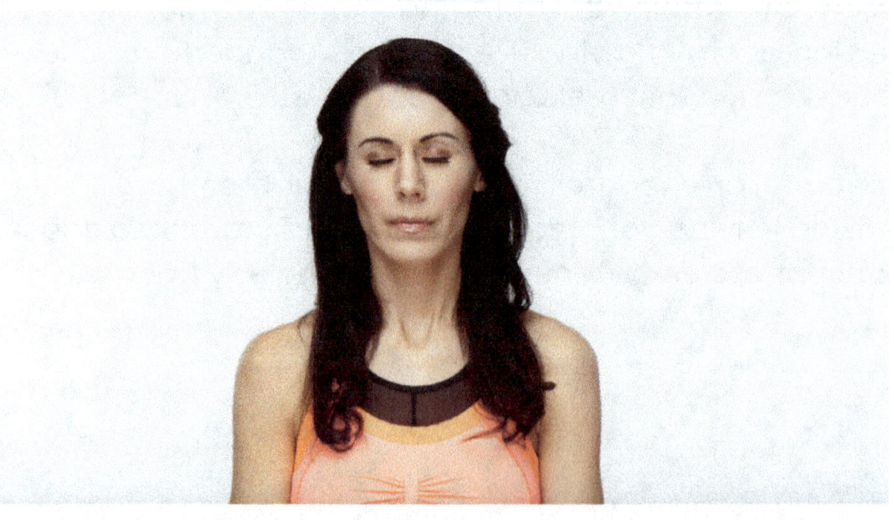

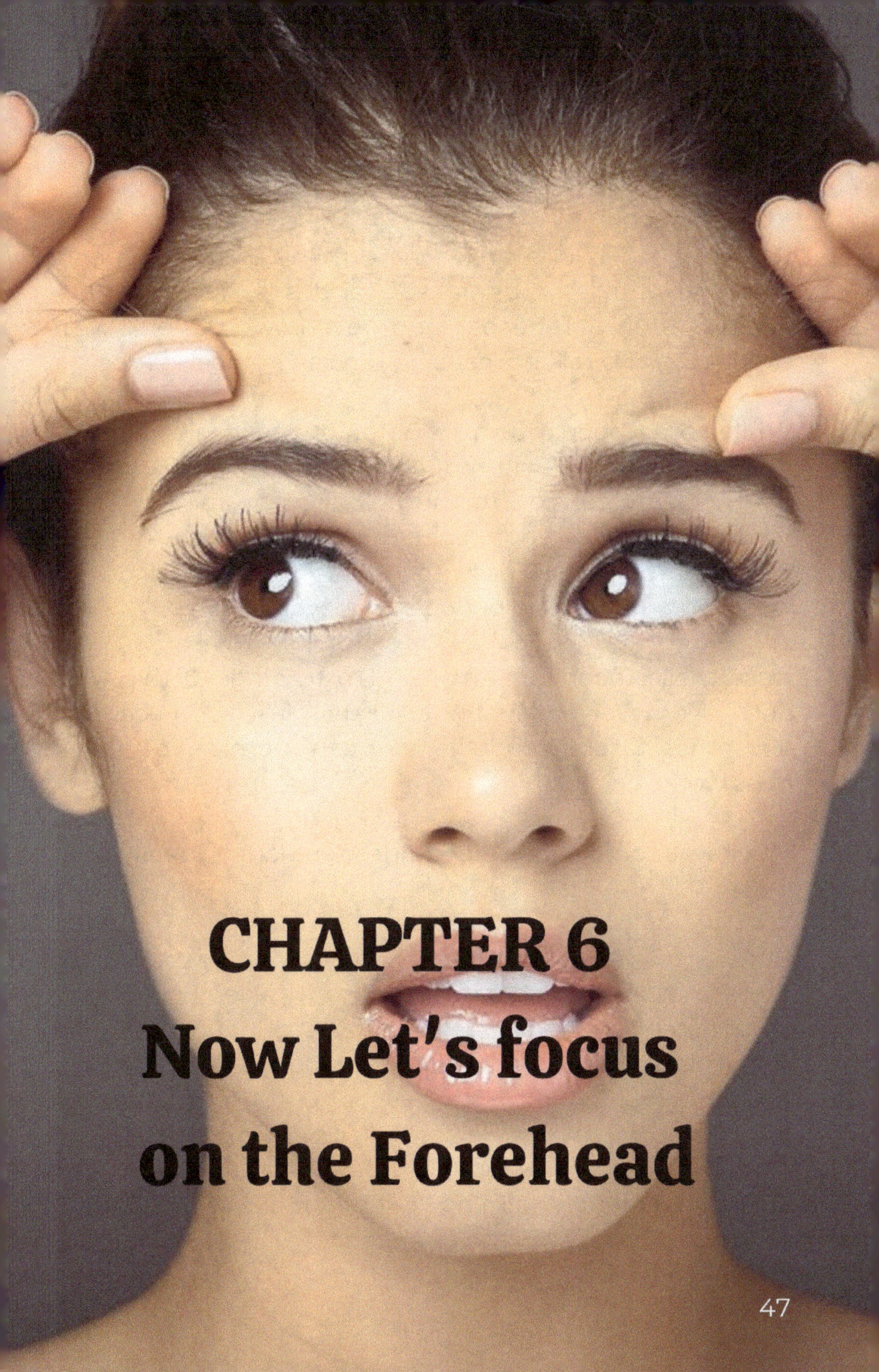

CHAPTER 6
Now Let's focus
on the Forehead

5 ways to reduce forehead lines without injectables

The forehead is one area where many of us experience lines and wrinkles. A big reason for this is that we tend to overuse our foreheads and eyebrows when we're expressing and talking, causing tension in the muscles.

While some people turn to Botox or other injectables to relax the forehead and reduce lines and wrinkles, we can easily release tension in the muscles naturally by using some simple Face Yoga techniques. In this post, I'm going to run through five easy techniques that focus on the forehead and the area between our eyebrows.

I use these techniques myself. I'm turning 40 this week and have never had Botox or fillers. I just use Face Yoga and other natural products, so I can promise you that it does work..

The key is to do these techniques regularly – ideally every day.

But if you already have forehead lines, don't worry. Firstly, there's nothing wrong with lines and wrinkles. Face yoga is all about helping you feel healthy and happy from the inside out so that your skin looks the best it can for the age you are.

This easy Face Yoga sequence takes less than ten minutes and is a beautifully calming routine to release tension and soothe the muscles in the forehead.

BEFORE YOU START

Make sure your hands and face are clean before you start any Face Yoga routine. We're focusing on massage techniques in this sequence, so it helps to apply a few drops of serum to help your fingers move easily over your skin.

I use my Fusion by Danielle Collins Pro Lift Facial Moisturising Serum. As well as giving a lovely glide while you're massaging your skin, this serum is packed full of high-performing botanical seed oils. It's non-greasy and won't block your pores, but it does penetrate into the middle layer of your skin, the dermis.

The dermis is where elastin and collagen are produced, so you'll be getting all those active, organic ingredients and nourishing vitamins to the area where you need them most. The serum is also vegan, organic, and certified by the Soil Association.

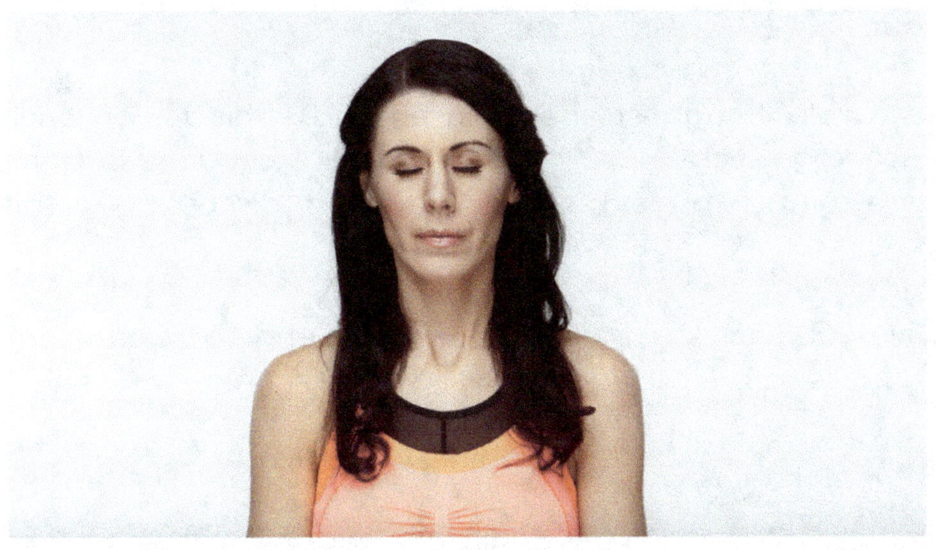

1. SMOOTH

Place your hands on your forehead and gently smooth outwards. Replace them at the centre and then repeat.

This technique is very simple, but it is also effective. It targets the frontalis muscle, which is the large one that covers most of the front of our foreheads.

Most of us overuse this muscle in day-to-day life and it ends up holding a lot of tension. This simple massage technique starts to relax the muscle, meaning we are less likely to overexpress with it and end up with lines and wrinkles.

The massage also boosts blood circulation, bringing fresh blood, oxygen, and nutrients up to the surface of your skin. This helps to brighten your skin too.

You don't need to press hard here to see the benefits. Just a gentle pressure is fine and feels beautifully soothing on your skin.

As a rule, I suggest spending around 1 minute on each Face Yoga technique. There are some exceptions but aim for a minute for each of the moves I'm discussing in this post.

Give your arms a little shake at the end to release any stiffness before moving on to the next technique.

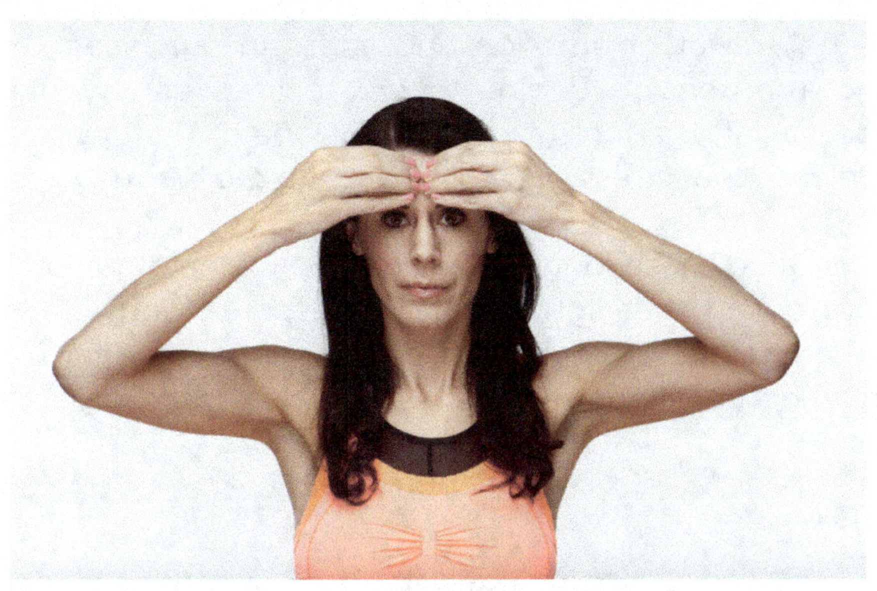

2. ARCHES

We're still working with the frontalis muscle for this next move. Take both your index fingers to your forehead, starting just above the inside corner of your eyebrows.

Draw your fingers up, across, and down, making an arch shape just above your eyebrows. Come back to your original starting point, but make the next arch slightly higher, crossing over the middle of your forehead. Your third arch should come right up to the top of your forehead

Go back to the beginning and repeat this sequence for around a minute.

As you continue with the massage, bring your attention to your breath. Take a deep inhale through your nose, feeling your abdomen rise. Then exhale long and slow, still through your nose. Let your abdomen drop down again.

We hold a lot of emotion and stress in our faces. Over time, this tension begins to create lines and wrinkles, especially in the forehead area. But one of the best ways to release that stress is to come back to the breath.

As we take these long, deep breaths, we help our brains move out of that fight-and-flight response and into our calmer, rest-and-digest state. Feeling calmer and less stressed also gives us a more relaxed, healthier face.

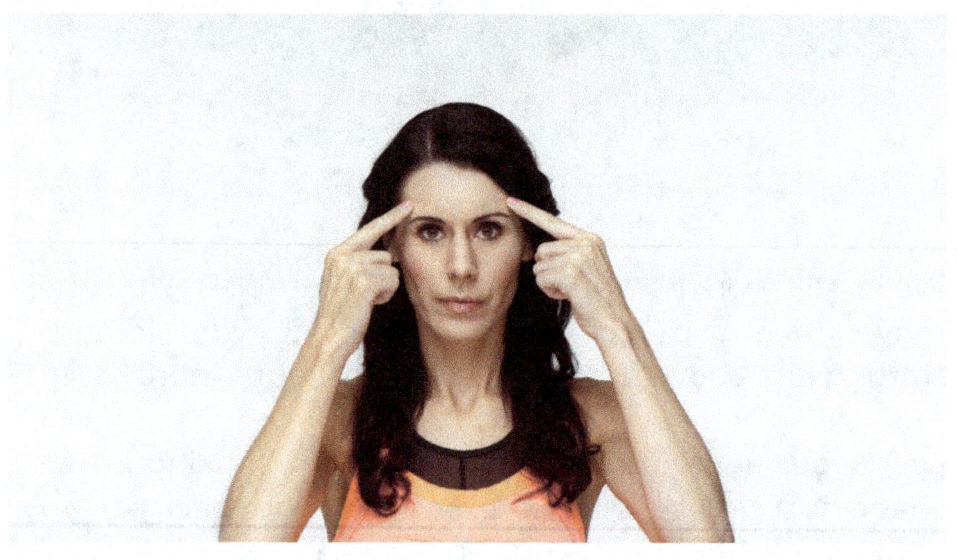

3. EYE MUSCLES

Place your hands on your forehead. Use your fingers to keep your eyebrows and forehead still as you open your eyes as wide as you can. Focus on a point straight in front of you.

The aim here is to engage the orbicularis oculi muscles, which go right around each eye. Try to keep the frontalis muscle at the front of the forehead still as you use the eye muscles to widen your eyes. Notice how it feels to use your eye muscles to express instead of your forehead.

Shake out your arms and close your eyes for a moment. Then take the pose again. This time, use your eyes to look right and left, holding the rest of your face still.

These eye movements have been used in yoga for thousands of years. They help to strengthen the muscles around the eyes, improving our eyesight at the same time as tightening and tautening the skin attached to the muscles.

Shake out your hands and then take the pose again. This time, use your eyes to look up and down while your hands keep your forehead as still as possible.

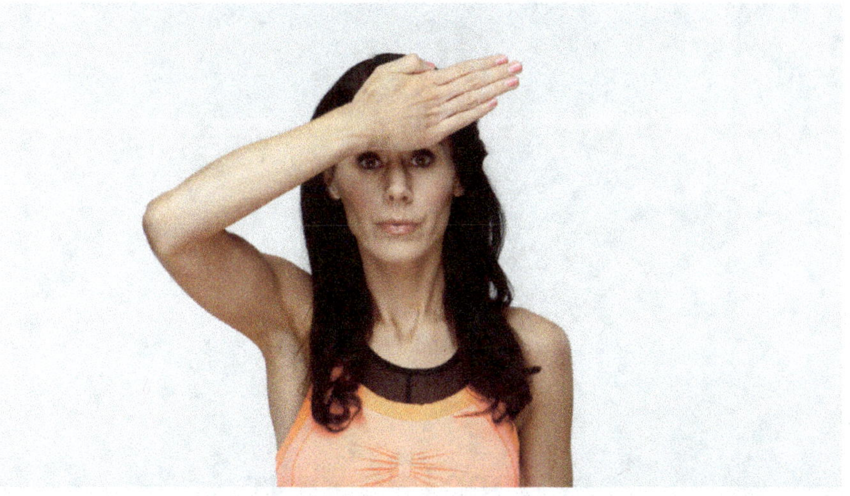

4. HOOK

This next technique targets the procerus muscle, which runs up between the eyebrows. This is another muscle that we tend to overuse when we express. But when we combine the breath with facial massage and focus on releasing this area, we can relax it naturally.

Form your index finger into a hook shape. Using the middle knuckle, stroke up between your eyebrows and over your forehead. You might also come out at a slight angle on some of the strokes, making sure to cover the whole muscle.

Again, you can keep the pressure gentle here. With any Face Yoga technique, I urge you to work to your own level and use your intuition to guide you.
Focus on letting go of tension and give the muscle permission to release any stress or tightness.

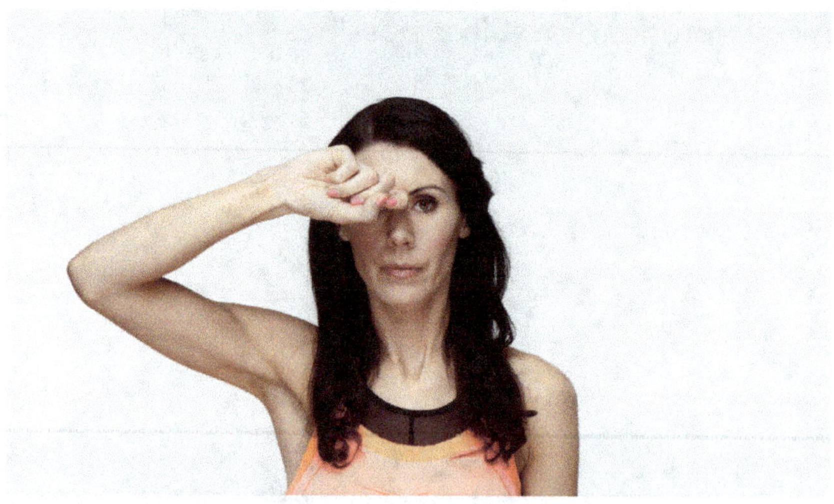

5. THIRD EYE POINT

Finally, place the tip of one index finger on the point between your eyebrows. Bring your attention back to your breath, taking long inhales and exhales through your nose as you press gently on this acupressure point.

This point is well-known in Ayurveda and Traditional Chinese Medicine for releasing stress and helping us to relax. It is called the third eye point and it relates to our intuition and inner knowledge.

Pressing here helps to relax the procerus muscle further. It is also a great point to use if you are struggling to sleep or are feeling anxious.

After pressing for a few breaths, start to massage the point with a small circular motion. Go one way and then the other.

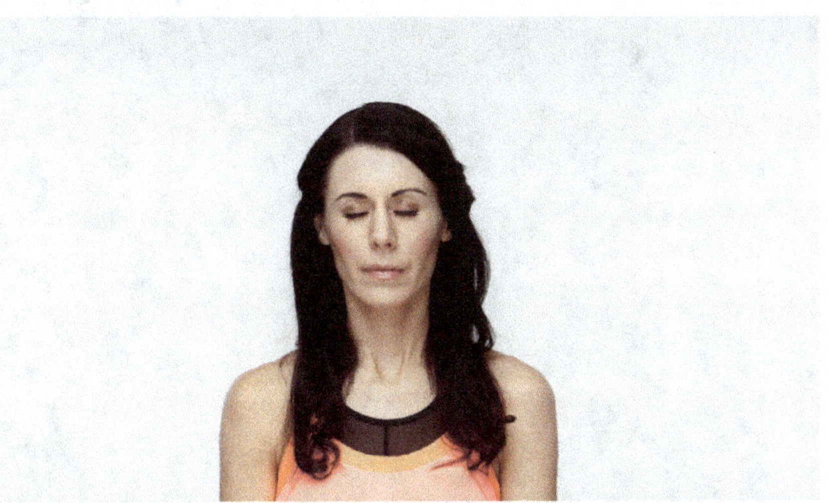

FINISHED

End the Face Yoga sequence by bringing your hands down and closing your eyes. Focus your attention on your forehead area and let go of any remaining tension. Visualise a white, healing light bathing the area as you take a few last deep breaths.

When you're ready, open your eyes. And we're all done!

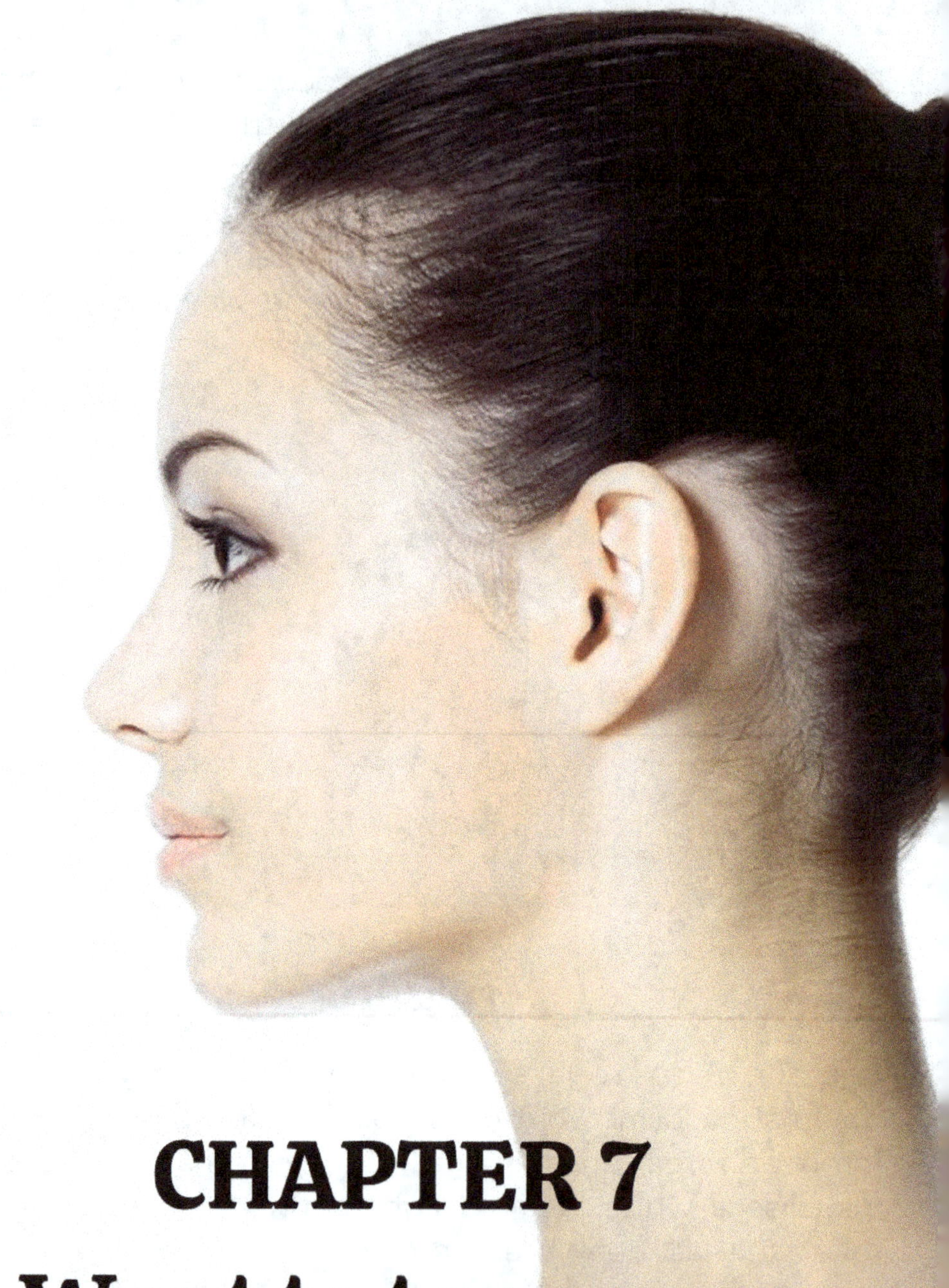

CHAPTER 7
Want to tone your Nose ?

Tone the Nose naturally with Face Yoga

ALTERNATE NOSE BREATHING

Step 1: Take your thumb and hold your left nostril closed — breath in with the other nostril.

Step 2: Hold both nostrils closed for 1 second and release your finger from your left nostril — exhaling at the release.

Step 3: Hold your right closed nostril with your index finger.

Step 4: Breath in through the opposite nostril.

Step 5: Hold both nostrils closed for one second and release.

Repeat this sequence for about 1 minute.

This exercise helps to tone the cartilage in the nostrils. It also aids in reducing anxiety, clearing sinuses, and balancing both brain hemispheres.

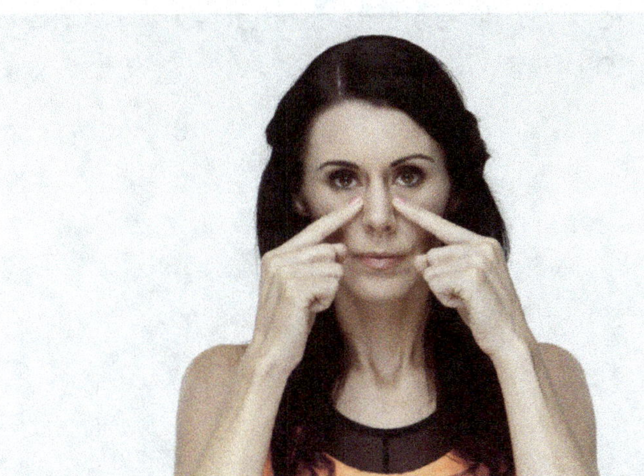

NASALIS TONING

Step 1: Place your two index fingers beside your nostrils.

Step 2: Press your fingers in this area — applying moderate pressure.

Step 3: Flare and release your nostrils against the resistance of your fingers at a rate of 1 'flare' per second.

Repeat this exercise for up to 1 minute.

This exercise helps to strengthen the nasalis muscle, which helps give the bridge of your nose a slimmed appearance.

NOSE TIP PRESS

Step 1: Place your index finger on the tip of your nose.

Step 2: Apply slight pressure, pressing downward.

Step 3: Take deep breaths in and out.

Repeat this exercise for up to 1 minute.

This exercise helps to keep the cartilage in the tip of your nose strong and healthy.

NOSE BRIDGE MASSAGE

Step 1: Place index and thumb on each side of your nose bridge.

Step 2: Applying slight pressure, gently massage the bridge of your nose — going in an up and down motion.

Repeat this exercise for up to 1 minute.

This technique boosts circulation in your skin and helps keep the area firm.

NASOLABIAL MASSAGE

Step 1: Tuck your lips inward — so that your mouth forms a straight line.

Step 2: Take your index finger and place them on the sides of your mouth — where your nasolabial folds are.

Step 3: Slightly lift the corners of your lips — making a smiling shape.

Step 4: Use index fingers to smooth the skin on the sides on the mouth

Repeat the massaging motion for up to 1 minute.
This face yoga technique helps to lift the cheeks and smooth out smile lines.

CHEEK TAP

Step 1: Puff out your cheeks.

Step 2: Using three fingers — index, middle, and ring finger — press down on top of your lips.

Step 3: Lightly tap your cheek — repeat this for 10 seconds and switch sides.

Alternate sides for 1 minute.

This exercise helps to tone cheek muscles and boost circulation in the skin surrounding your nose.

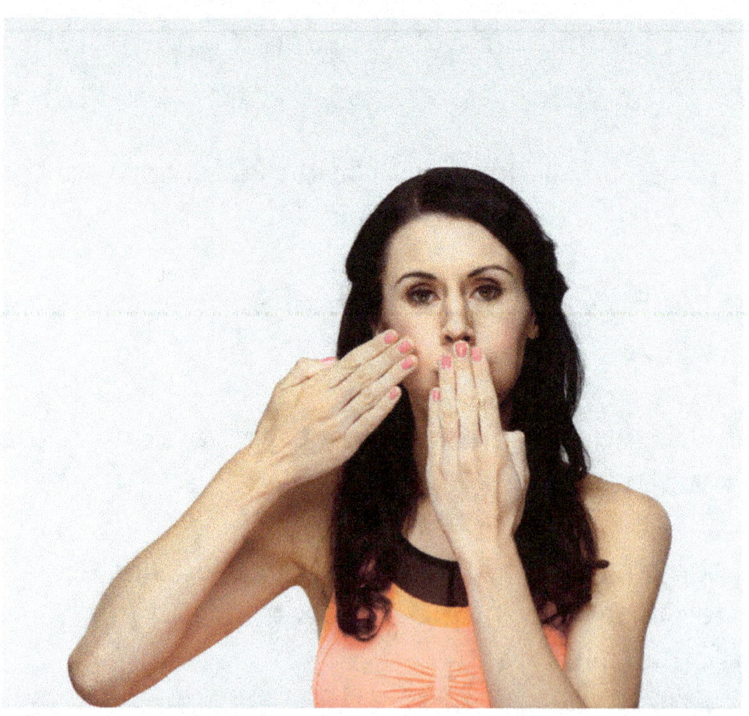

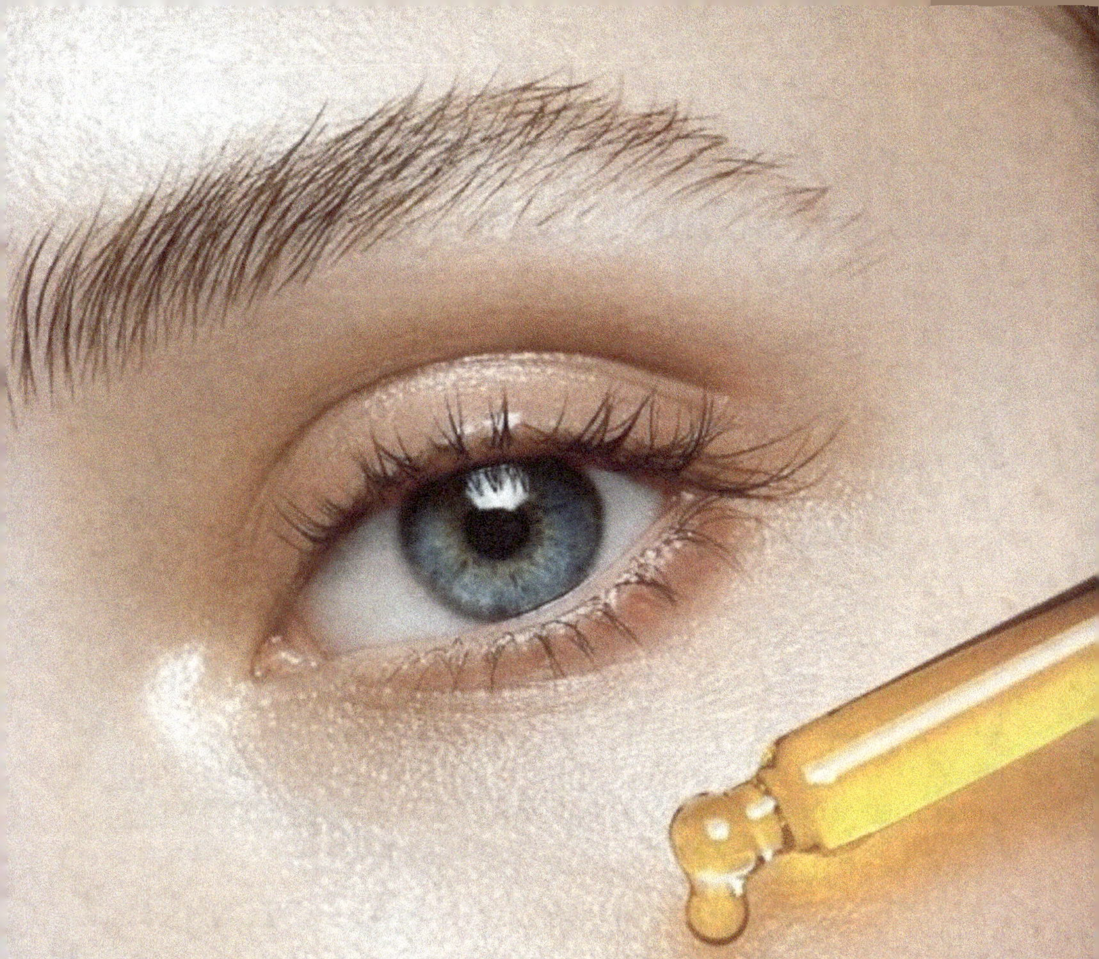

CHAPTER 8
Last but not least...
It's time for your
Eyes

5 Face Yoga moves to reduce malar bags/festoons/under eye swelling

Malar bags, or festoons, are a common form of under-eye swelling that many of us start to develop as we get older. They are a bit different from puffiness, which usually appears directly under the lower eyelids. You'll usually find the swelling associated with malar bags or festoons lower down, across the top of your cheekbones.

In this post, I'm running through a simple Face Yoga routine to reduce or prevent malar bags without needing to resort to surgery. In total, it should take just ten minutes, so you can hopefully make it part of your daily routine without too much difficulty.

WHAT CAUSES MALAR BAGS AND FESTOONS?

Many different factors can affect whether we develop malar bags and other forms of swelling under the eyes. Most of these are to do with lifestyle.

Sun damage is a really big one. In fact, around 80% of skin ageing is caused by sun exposure, so it is vital that you make sure you are applying your SPF every single day. It is one of the best things you can do to protect your skin. This includes on cloudy days or when you are going to be inside – those harmful UVA rays penetrate through glass too.

Other lifestyle factors that can affect your risk of developing malar bags or festoons include:
- Your stress levels
- Your sleep

- Your diet
- Your alcohol consumption
- Smoking

Age also plays a big part. As we get older, the natural loss of collagen and elastin from the dermis (middle layer of skin) leaves us more prone to swelling.

There's also a genetic component. But don't worry – even if your parents or grandparents had malar bags, it doesn't mean you'll definitely get them too. Making the right lifestyle choices really helps to reduce swelling and can even prevent it altogether.

BEFORE YOU START

Make sure you have clean hands and a clean face before you begin this face yoga routine.

Apply a few drops of the Fusion by Danielle Collins Serum to the area above your cheekbones. This helps your fingers to glide easily over the skin without dragging. It is also packed with high-performing botanical seed oils designed to nourish your skin.

Unlike most creams and moisturisers, the molecules in this serum are small enough to penetrate into the middle layer of your skin, the dermis. This is where collagen and elastin production takes place. As a result, you'll get all the vital vitamins from the organic seed oils deep into your skin.
I like to use the serum in place of a moisturiser.

It is non-greasy and won't block your pores. But I know other people prefer to layer it under their regular moisturiser. Either way works!

1. LYMPHATIC MASSAGE

Place the tips of your ring fingers at the inside corners of your eyes. Keeping your touch very light, smooth your fingers up beneath your eyebrows, across to the outer corners, and then down over the tops of your cheeks.

Continue with this circular massage for a minute or two, concentrating on the area where you notice the swelling. As you massage, connect with your breath. Feel your abdomen rise and fall as you take deep, slow inhales and exhales through your nose.

It is important to work very gently around the eyes. The skin here is thin and delicate, so we don't want to drag or pull at it. Applying serum will help your fingers to move easily.

You might feel like you're not doing much here. But there's no need to be heavy-handed, especially when we're working with lymphatic drainage. In fact, going gently will give you better results.

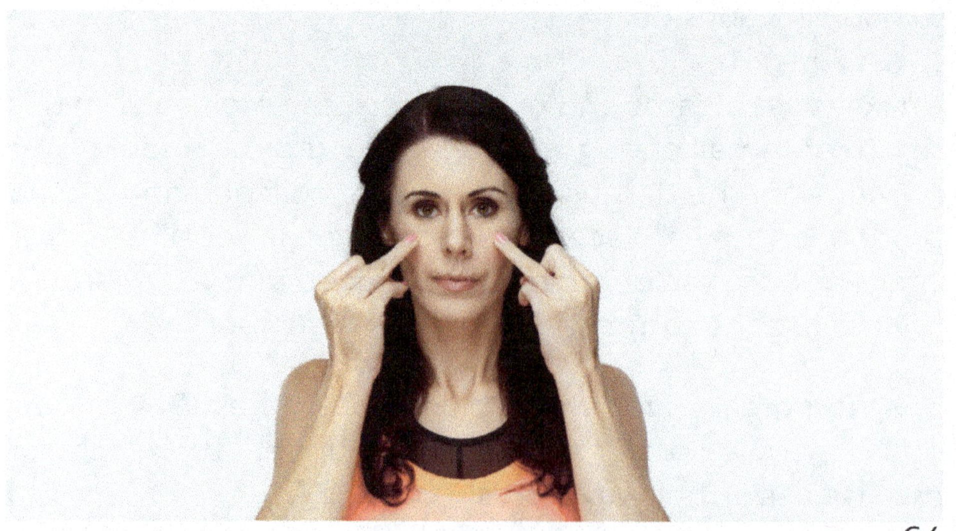

2. PULSE

Next, take three fingers underneath each eye where the swelling is. Press gently – again, there's no need to go too hard here.

Gently pulse your fingers to stimulate the lymphatic drainage further. Continue for a minute or two.

Remember to keep those deep, calming breaths going as you pulse. Try to relax the rest of your face too.

This technique also helps to relieve puffiness and dark circles.

3. FLIRTY EYES

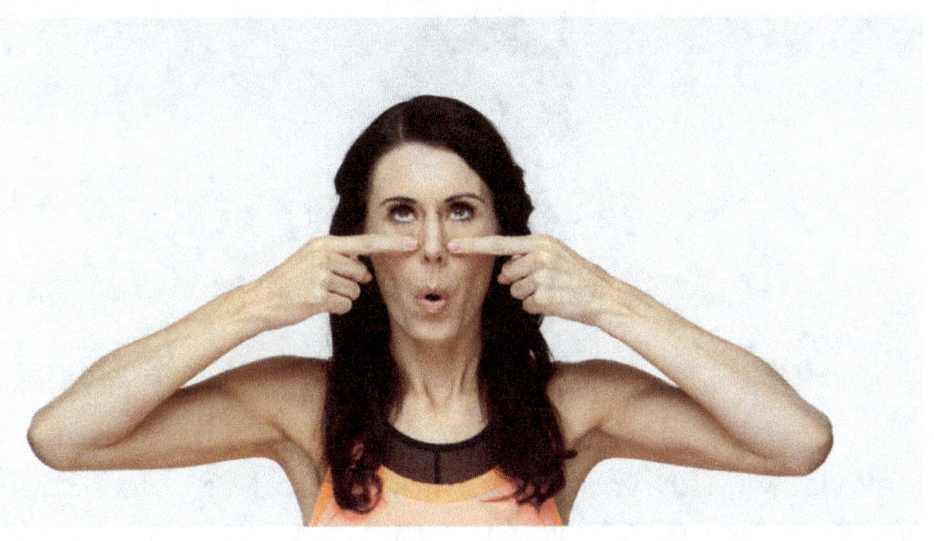

Place your index fingers horizontally beneath your eyes where the swelling occurs. Your fingertips should rest near your nose. Your fingers are mainly there to provide some resistance and engage the muscles further.

Make an 'O' shape with your mouth, tucking your lips around your teeth. Moving just your eyes, look up towards the ceiling. Flutter your upper eyelids rapidly for around 45 seconds.

Close your eyes for a moment and take a deep breath in and out through your nose. Tune into how your eye area is feeling. Hopefully, you will already notice the lifeforce running freely instead of being blocked or stagnant. Known as prana in yoga or Chi in Traditional Chinese Medicine, this energy helps to reduce lines, wrinkles, and swelling.

4. V / MINI-V

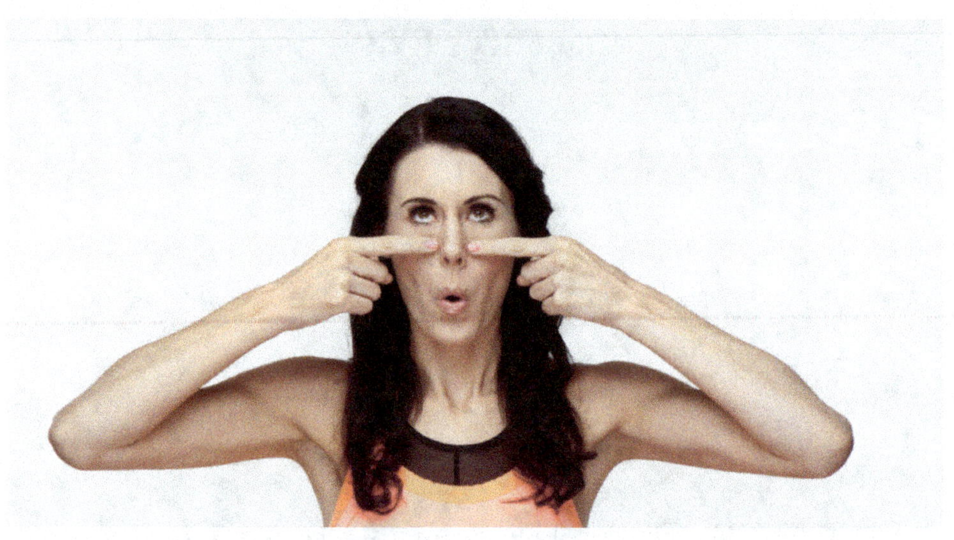

Make a 'V' with your index fingers and middle fingers. There are two variations of this move.

You place the middle fingers between your eyebrows and the index fingers at the outer edge of your eyes. This works a bit more of the muscle, so I recommend this variation if you have quite pronounced malar bags or festoons.

In this variation, you place your fingers lower down. The middle finger sits at the inner corner of your eye.

This works less of the muscle but gets deeper. I suggest trying this version if your swelling is closer to the eye, or if you are prone to crows' feet.

Look up towards the ceiling. Half-close your eyes, feeling for a little flutter in the muscle underneath your index finger. Hold for two to three seconds, then release. Take the pose again, repeating it five times in total.

Don't worry if you don't feel that little flutter at first. It takes some practice to get the hang of this technique.

5. DRAINING THE LYMPH

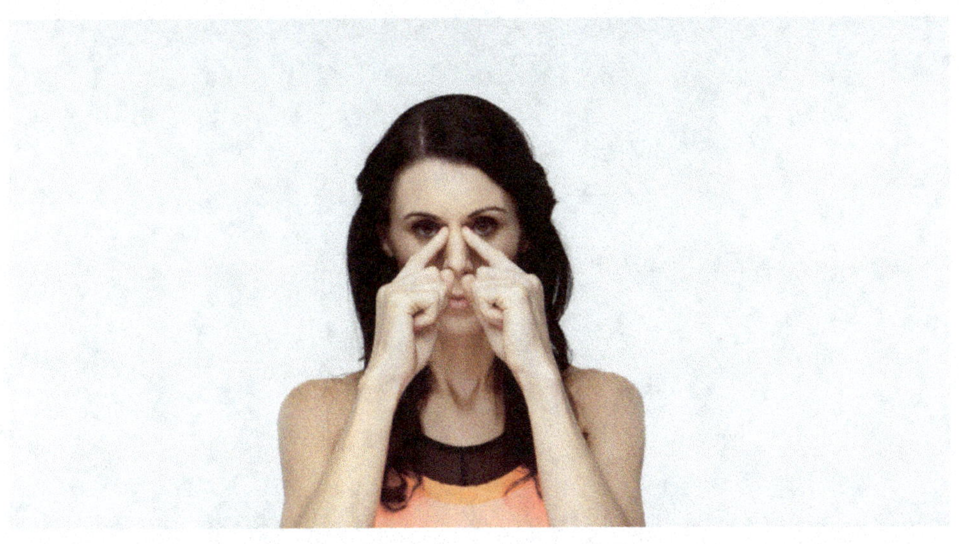

Our final move returns to working with lymphatic drainage. Take your index fingers to the acupressure point at the inner corner of your eyes. Keeping your touch as light as a feather, glide your fingers over the swollen area.

Continue smoothing over the sides of your face to your temples and then go around behind the ears and down the sides of your neck until you reach your collarbone.

Repeat several times to help to drain fluid away from your eye area and reduce swelling.

FINISHED!

And that's it. Hopefully, your eye area already feels refreshed and energised.

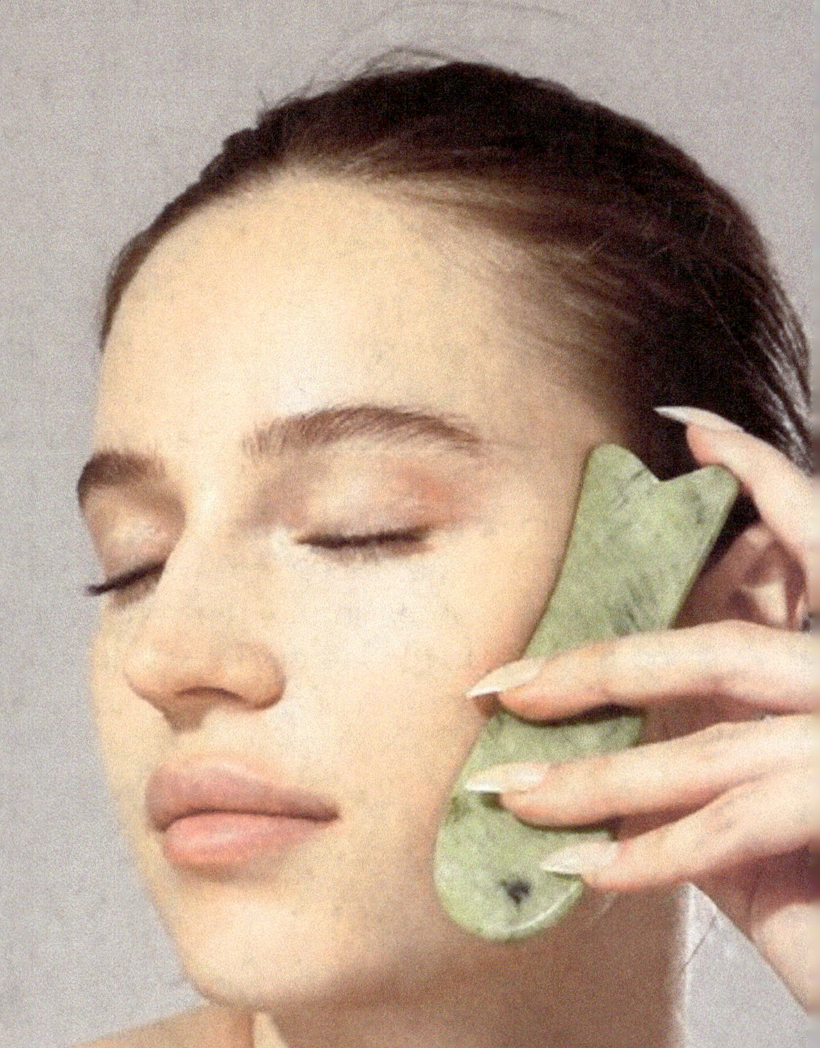

CHAPTER 9
How to use a gua sha for beginners

How to use a gua sha for beginners

If you're interested in holistic and natural approaches to skincare, I'm sure you will have heard of Gua Sha – it has become increasingly popular over the last few years (for good reason).

It's also something I talk about a lot because Gua Sha is a wonderful complement to face yoga. It comes from Traditional Chinese Medicine and is a form of massage that is usually done with a tool made from crystal.

As a beginner, it can be difficult to know where to start with Gua Sha to get the best results, so this blog will walk you through some simple techniques you can use to smooth the skin, reduce puffiness and inflammation, and leave your face looking bright, lifted, and toned.

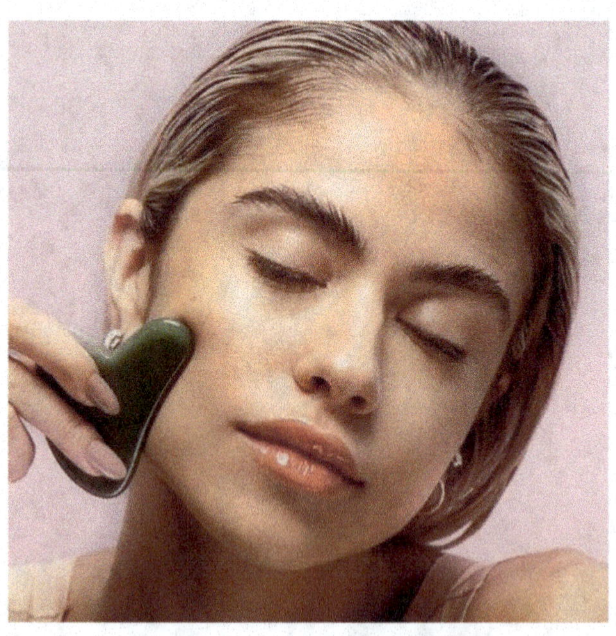

GETTING STARTED

First, make sure you have a clean face and clean hands before starting your Gua Sha routine. Then, apply a few drops of serum to help the tool glide over your skin. I use the Fusion by Danielle Collins Pro Lift Moisturising Serum, which is specifically designed for use with face yoga and facial massage techniques, including Gua Sha.

You can use which ever Gua Sha crystal you feel intuitively drawn too. If you have sensitive or more mature skin or you know you'll be doing Gua Sha mainly in the morning, you might opt for a rose quartz Gua Sha tool. Alternatively, if you'll be doing Gua Sha mainly in the evening or are looking to soothe away stress, then you might find a clear quartz Gua Sha tool works best for you.

Of course, you may eventually have multiple tools so that you can vary depending on your skin's needs, but as a beginner you just want to choose the one that feels right for you to start with.

Final thing before we start with some techniques; Gua Sha is a beautiful form of face massage and is suitable for most skin types. However, if you are in the first trimester of pregnancy, have recently had Botox or fillers, or have any easily aggravated skin conditions, please consult a medical professional before using Gua Sha.

If none of this applies to you, then you should be good to go. Just remember to always work to your own level, as with any of my face yoga or facial massage routines.

1. PRESS AND HOLD

We're going to start by simply pressing the flat surface of the Gua Sha tool against the skin, with the S-shaped edge facing up and resting just beneath your eye. The rest of the tool presses against your cheek.

This is a gentle way to soothe the skin, reducing puffiness around the eye area. You can make the effect even more soothing by keeping your Gua Sha in the fridge.

I also like to press and hold the tool across my forehead, on my cheeks, and against my jawline.

2. LYMPHATIC DRAINAGE

One of the major benefits of Gua Sha is that it stimulates lymphatic drainage, helping to move waste away from your face. This leaves your skin looking brighter and healthier, as well as reducing puffiness.

Using the long concave edge of the tool, lightly stroke down the sides of your neck, starting just behind your earlobe and finishing at your collarbone. Give the tool a little wiggle when you reach your collarbone, then come back up and repeat a couple more times before moving to the other side.

Keep your Gua Sha tool at a 10–45-degree angle with your skin as you move it.

3. JAW

Next, use the S-shaped edge of the tool to smooth along your jaw, starting at your chin and working out towards your ear. Repeat a few times.

I like to place my index finger on the outer corner of my jaw while I do this move to hold the skin taut and prevent any dragging.

This is great for releasing jaw tension and lifting and sculpting the jawline. Make sure you repeat on the other side too.

4. CHEEKS

Remembering to hold the tool at a 10 – 45-degree angle, use the long concave edge to smooth across your cheeks. You want to hold the tool vertically and move it in an upward swoosh, working out from your nose and following the curve of your cheekbone.

Again, if you find your skin is getting dragged a bit, you can use your other hand near your ear to hold it taut while you do this technique.

You'll probably notice some redness (Sha) coming up on your skin – this is a great sign!

Gua Sha is designed to boost blood circulation as well as lymphatic drainage, so the redness indicates increased blood flow to your skin. It will quickly fade once you finish the sequence.

5. EYE AREA

Next, use the rounded corner where the S-shaped edge meets the concave edge to massage around your eye area. Start at the inner corner of your eye, then gently move down, under the eye, and up to your temple.

This is lovely for reducing puffiness and dark circles under the eyes.

6. FOREHEAD

Starting in the centre of your forehead, stroke outwards three to six times, using the concave edge of the tool. Repeat on the other side to smooth the skin.

Then, take the S-shaped edge and stroke upwards between your eyes. This is an area that often holds a lot of tension, so this technique really helps to release some of that, increase blood flow, and reduce number 11 lines.

FINISH

Finish off your Gua Sha sequence by repeating the long strokes down the side of your neck that we did in step 2.

This is just a taster of the many techniques that you can do with a Gua Sha tool. For example, you can also use the rounded corners on your acupressure points for a little acupressure massage. There are warm-up and cool-down techniques, moves for lifting and sculpting, routines focusing on lymphatic drainage, and more.

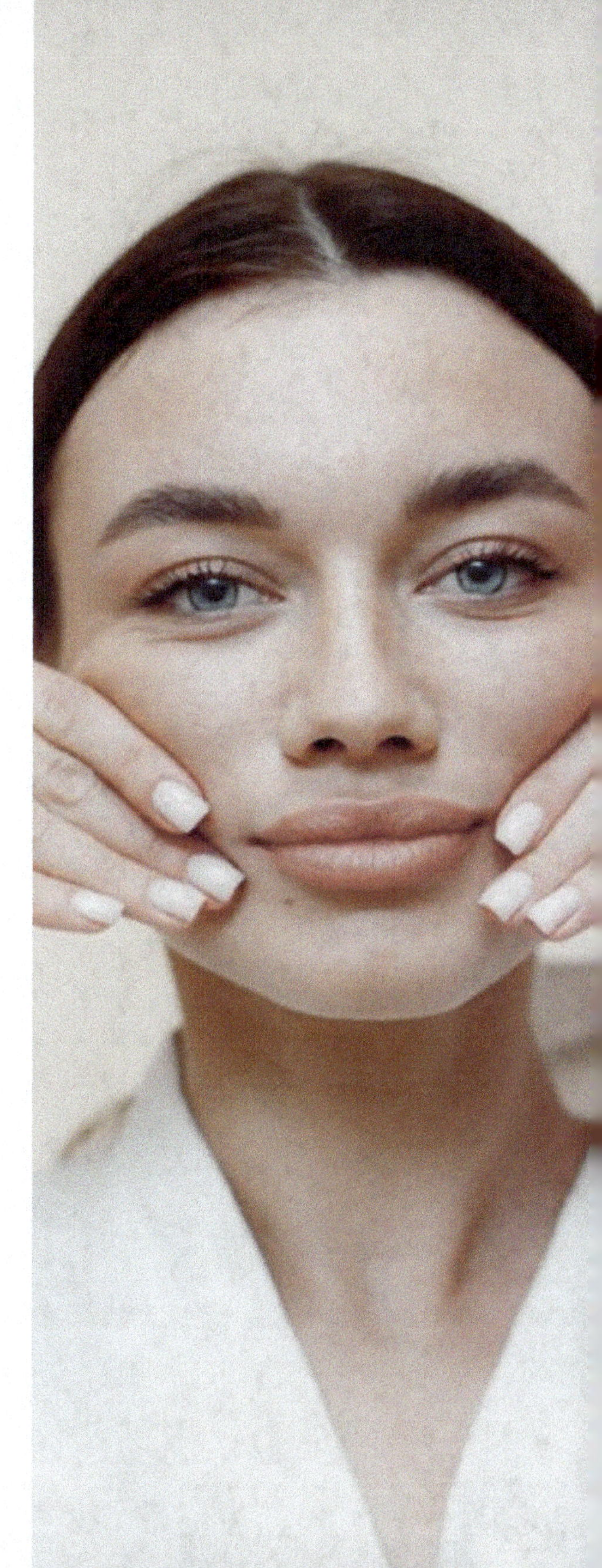

Thank You For Reading!